Unveiling Strength: A Compassionate Guide Through the Cancer Journey for Moms

Table of Contents: Cancer Journey for Moms

Introduction

The journey through cancer is a formidable challenge, one that requires courage, resilience, and a strong support system. For moms facing this journey, the complexities are heightened as they navigate the delicate balance of caring for themselves while continuing to nurture and support their families. This guide is crafted with a deep understanding of the unique challenges that mothers encounter when confronted with a cancer diagnosis.

In this introductory section, we'll set the stage for the exploration of the cancer journey for moms, emphasizing the importance of support, both from loved ones and the broader community. We'll provide an overview of what the journey entails, acknowledging the emotional and practical hurdles that moms may encounter along the way. As we delve into the subsequent chapters, our goal is to empower moms with knowledge, practical strategies, and emotional resilience to face the path ahead. Remember, you are not alone—countless others have walked a similar road, and together, we can find strength, hope, and healing.

Overview of the Cancer Journey

The cancer journey is a profound and transformative experience that touches every aspect of a person's life. For moms, this expedition carries unique challenges, intertwining their roles as caregivers with the demands of their own health. Understanding the broader context of the cancer journey is essential to navigate its twists and turns with resilience and grace.

The Uncharted Terrain

The initial shock of a cancer diagnosis often plunges individuals and their families into uncharted terrain. This section explores the emotional impact of receiving such news, addressing the fear, uncertainty, and the myriad of questions that arise. For moms, the added concern for the well-being of their children and family amplifies the complexities of this initial phase.

The Medical Landscape

This subsection provides an overview of the medical aspects of the cancer journey, from diagnostic procedures to treatment modalities. Understanding the language of oncology, the significance of various tests, and the available treatment options empowers moms to actively participate in decision-making processes regarding their healthcare.

The Role of Support

Navigating the cancer journey is not a solitary endeavor. It requires a robust support system. Here, we delve into the vital role that family, friends, and community can play in providing emotional, practical, and moral support for moms. We'll explore the importance of effective communication and building a network that fosters strength and resilience.

A Holistic Approach

The cancer journey extends beyond medical treatments; it encompasses the mental, emotional, and physical well-being of individuals. This section introduces the concept of a holistic approach, emphasizing the importance of addressing not only the disease itself but also the overall health and quality of life of moms on this journey.

Importance of Support for Moms

Cancer is not a battle meant to be fought alone, and for moms facing this formidable challenge, a robust support system is not just beneficial—it's essential. In this section, we delve into the profound impact that emotional, practical, and social support can have on the well-being of moms navigating the complexities of a cancer journey.

Emotional Support: Nurturing the Spirit

The emotional toll of a cancer diagnosis is significant, and moms, in their roles as caregivers, may grapple with a unique set of emotions. Here, we explore the importance of emotional support, whether through empathetic conversations with loved ones, counseling services, or support groups. Understanding and processing these emotions is a crucial aspect of maintaining mental well-being throughout the journey.

Practical Support: Easing the Burden

Cancer treatment often brings about practical challenges, from managing appointments and medications to juggling household responsibilities. This subsection outlines the practical aspects of support, including organizing help from friends and family, accessing community resources, and finding assistance for daily tasks. By alleviating some of the logistical burdens, moms can focus more on their health and recovery.

Social Support: Building a Community

The power of community cannot be overstated. This section explores the importance of building a social support network for moms facing cancer. Whether through local support groups, online communities, or connecting with other moms who have experienced similar journeys, the shared wisdom and camaraderie can provide a sense of belonging and encouragement.

The Role of Partners and Family

Partners and family members play a central role in the support structure for moms dealing with cancer. We discuss strategies for open communication, mutual understanding, and the ways in which partners and family members can actively contribute to creating a nurturing environment.

Professional Support: Healthcare Teams and Beyond

Beyond personal networks, professional support is a cornerstone of the cancer journey. This subsection emphasizes the importance of a collaborative relationship with healthcare professionals, including oncologists, nurses, and support staff. Additionally, we explore complementary support services such as social workers, therapists, and nutritionists who can contribute to a holistic approach to well-being.

Chapter 1: Understanding Cancer

Cancer is a complex group of diseases characterized by the uncontrolled growth and spread of abnormal cells. To navigate the challenges of a cancer journey, it is essential for moms to have a foundational understanding of the disease. In this section, we explore the basics of cancer, including its types, causes, risk factors, and the importance of early detection.

Types of Cancer

Cancer manifests in various forms, each with its unique characteristics and treatment approaches. This subsection provides an overview of common types of cancer that affect women, addressing breast cancer, ovarian cancer, uterine cancer, and others. Understanding the specific type of cancer is crucial for tailoring treatment plans and making informed decisions.

Causes and Risk Factors

Cancer arises from a combination of genetic, environmental, and lifestyle factors. Here, we delve into the causes of cancer, exploring genetic mutations, exposure to carcinogens, and lifestyle choices that may contribute to the development of the disease. Moms will gain insights into risk factors and how certain factors may increase or decrease the likelihood of cancer.

Early Detection and Screening

Early detection plays a pivotal role in improving cancer outcomes. This subsection emphasizes the significance of regular screenings and diagnostic tests for moms, guiding them on when and how to undergo screenings based on their age, family history, and other risk factors. Knowledge of early detection methods empowers moms to take a proactive approach to their health.

The Cancer Journey: From Diagnosis to Treatment

Understanding the trajectory of the cancer journey is essential for moms facing a diagnosis. We explore the diagnostic process, including imaging, biopsies, and pathology reports. Additionally, this section provides an overview of various treatment modalities, such as surgery, chemotherapy, radiation therapy, and immunotherapy. Moms will gain insights into the potential side effects and challenges associated with each treatment option.

Hormonal Factors

Hormonal changes and imbalances can contribute to the development of specific cancers, particularly those affecting the reproductive system. This section discusses how factors such as hormone replacement therapy, oral contraceptives, and pregnancy can influence cancer risk. Moms will gain insights into managing hormonal factors in consultation with healthcare professionals.

Age and Gender

Cancer risk often increases with age, and certain types of cancer may exhibit gender-specific patterns. Here, we explore how age and gender play a role in cancer incidence, emphasizing the importance of age-appropriate screenings and awareness. Moms will gain insights into age-related considerations and how to stay vigilant about their health at different life stages.

Immunodeficiency and Chronic Conditions

Individuals with weakened immune systems or certain chronic conditions may face an elevated risk of developing cancer. This subsection explores the relationship between immunodeficiency, chronic illnesses, and cancer risk. Moms with underlying health conditions will gain insights into managing their overall health in collaboration with healthcare professionals.

Early Detection and Screening

Early detection is a cornerstone of effective cancer management, significantly improving treatment outcomes and survival rates. For moms navigating the complexities of a cancer journey, understanding the importance of early detection and engaging in regular screenings is paramount. In this section, we explore various screening methods and emphasize the proactive steps moms can take to detect cancer in its early, more treatable stages.

Breast Cancer Screening

Breast cancer screening is crucial for early detection, and moms will learn about the importance of regular breast self-exams, clinical breast exams, and mammograms. This subsection provides guidance on when and how to perform self-exams, what to expect during clinical exams, and the role of mammography in detecting abnormalities.

Cervical Cancer Screening

Regular screenings, including Pap smears and HPV tests, are vital for detecting cervical cancer in its early stages. This section discusses the frequency of screenings, the significance of Pap smear results, and the role of HPV vaccination in preventing cervical cancer. Moms will gain insights into the proactive steps they can take to safeguard their cervical health.

Colorectal Cancer Screening

Colorectal cancer screenings, such as colonoscopies and stool tests, are essential for detecting abnormalities in the colon or rectum. This subsection explores the different screening methods, their recommended frequencies, and the importance of early detection in improving outcomes. Moms will gain a comprehensive understanding of how to navigate colorectal cancer screenings.

Ovarian Cancer Awareness

Early detection of ovarian cancer poses unique challenges, as symptoms are often subtle. This section discusses the importance of recognizing potential symptoms, such as bloating and pelvic pain, and seeking prompt medical attention. Moms will gain insights into the role of imaging tests and blood tests in aiding the early detection of ovarian cancer.

Lung Cancer Screening

For moms at risk of lung cancer, particularly those with a history of smoking, regular screenings using imaging tests can aid in early detection. This subsection explores the criteria for lung cancer screening, the role of computed tomography (CT) scans, and the importance of discussing screening options with healthcare providers.

Skin Cancer Checks

Skin cancer screenings involve regular self-exams and professional checks by dermatologists. This section provides guidance on recognizing changes in moles or skin lesions, practicing sun safety, and seeking professional dermatological assessments. Moms will gain insights into maintaining skin health and detecting potential signs of skin cancer early.

Regular Health Check-ups

Routine health check-ups play a pivotal role in overall cancer prevention and early detection. This subsection emphasizes the importance of regular visits to healthcare providers, where comprehensive health assessments and screenings can identify potential health concerns before they escalate.

Chapter 2: Diagnosis and Treatment

The journey through cancer involves a comprehensive process of diagnosis and subsequent treatment. For moms facing a cancer diagnosis, understanding the diagnostic procedures and treatment options is crucial. In this section, we explore the steps involved in the diagnosis of cancer and the various treatment modalities available, empowering moms to make informed decisions about their healthcare.

The Diagnostic Process

The journey begins with an accurate diagnosis. This subsection provides insights into the diagnostic procedures moms may undergo, including imaging tests, biopsies, and laboratory analyses. Understanding the diagnostic process is essential for moms to actively participate in discussions with healthcare professionals, ask informed questions, and comprehend the results.

Interpreting Diagnostic Results

Upon receiving diagnostic results, moms may face a spectrum of emotions and questions. This section guides them in interpreting test results, understanding medical terminologies, and seeking clarification from healthcare providers. The goal is to empower moms to be proactive partners in their healthcare journey, fostering open communication with the medical team.

Treatment Options

Cancer treatment is personalized and may involve a combination of modalities. This subsection explores various treatment options available to moms, including:

- Surgery: Understanding the role of surgical procedures in removing tumors and addressing cancer.
- Chemotherapy: Exploring the use of drugs to destroy cancer cells throughout the body.
- Radiation Therapy: Discussing the targeted use of high-dose radiation to eliminate cancer cells.
- Immunotherapy: Explaining how immunotherapy harnesses the body's immune system to fight cancer.
- Hormone Therapy: Addressing treatments that modify hormone levels to control certain types of cancer.
- Targeted Therapies: Exploring medications that target specific molecules involved in cancer growth.

Side Effects and Coping Strategies

Each treatment modality comes with its own set of side effects, impacting moms both physically and emotionally. This section discusses common side effects and provides practical strategies for managing them. From nausea and fatigue to emotional well-being, moms will find guidance on coping mechanisms and support systems to enhance their quality of life during treatment.

Integrative Therapies

Complementary and integrative therapies can play a supportive role in cancer treatment. This subsection explores approaches such as acupuncture, massage, yoga, and mindfulness, emphasizing their potential benefits in alleviating side effects and improving overall well-being. Moms will gain insights into incorporating these therapies into their treatment plans in consultation with healthcare providers.

The Diagnostic Process

Receiving a cancer diagnosis involves a thorough and systematic diagnostic process that aims to identify the type, stage, and extent of the disease. This section guides moms through the essential steps of the diagnostic journey, providing insights into the various tests and procedures they may encounter.

Initial Consultation and Medical History

The diagnostic process often begins with an in-depth consultation with a healthcare professional. Moms will learn about the importance of providing a detailed medical history, including family history, previous health issues, and any concerning symptoms. This initial discussion lays the foundation for the subsequent diagnostic steps.

Physical Examination

A comprehensive physical examination is a key component of the diagnostic process. Moms will gain an understanding of what to expect during a physical exam, including palpation of specific areas, examination of lymph nodes, and other relevant assessments. This step helps healthcare professionals identify potential signs of cancer.

Imaging Tests

Imaging tests play a crucial role in visualizing internal structures and detecting abnormalities. This subsection explores common imaging modalities such as X-rays, CT scans, MRIs, and PET scans. Moms will learn about the purposes of each test and what to expect during the procedures.

Biopsy and Pathology

When suspicious areas are identified through imaging, a biopsy may be recommended. This section explains the biopsy process, where a small sample of tissue is collected for examination. Understanding the role of pathology in analyzing biopsy samples helps moms grasp the intricacies of confirming a cancer diagnosis and determining its specific characteristics.

Laboratory Tests

Laboratory tests, including blood tests and tumor markers, provide valuable information about the overall health of moms and specific aspects of their cancer. This subsection discusses the significance of various blood parameters and tumor markers in the diagnostic process.

Staging and Grading

Once a cancer diagnosis is confirmed, healthcare professionals determine the stage and grade of the cancer. Moms will learn about the significance of staging in understanding the extent of the disease and guiding treatment decisions. Grading, which assesses the aggressiveness of the cancer cells, is also explained.

Second Opinion

Seeking a second opinion is a valuable step in the diagnostic process. Moms are encouraged to understand the importance of consulting with another healthcare professional to confirm the diagnosis, explore treatment options, and gain additional perspectives on their situation.

Treatment Options

Once a cancer diagnosis is confirmed, moms are faced with various treatment options tailored to their specific type and stage of cancer. Understanding these options empowers them to actively participate in decision-making alongside their healthcare team. This section explores the diverse modalities available for cancer treatment, addressing the goals, procedures, and potential side effects associated with each.

Surgery

Surgery is a common treatment option for many types of cancer. This subsection delves into the role of surgery in removing tumors, analyzing lymph nodes, and addressing cancerous tissue. Moms will gain insights into the pre-operative and post-operative processes, potential side effects, and the importance of discussing surgical options with their healthcare team.

Chemotherapy

Chemotherapy involves the use of drugs to target and kill rapidly dividing cancer cells. This section explores the various forms of chemotherapy, including intravenous infusions, oral medications, and combination therapies. Moms will learn about the treatment schedule, potential side effects such as nausea and fatigue, and strategies for managing these effects.

Radiation Therapy

Radiation therapy utilizes high-dose radiation to destroy or damage cancer cells. This subsection discusses the different types of radiation therapy, the treatment planning process, and potential side effects such as skin changes and fatigue. Moms will gain insights into the role of radiation therapy in various cancer types and its integration into a comprehensive treatment plan.

Immunotherapy

Immunotherapy harnesses the body's immune system to recognize and attack cancer cells. This section explores the different forms of immunotherapy, including checkpoint inhibitors and CAR-T cell therapy. Moms will learn about the potential side effects and the promising role of immunotherapy in treating certain cancers.

Hormone Therapy

Hormone therapy is used to modify hormone levels in the body, often for cancers that are hormone-sensitive. This subsection discusses how hormone therapy works, its applications in breast and ovarian cancers, and potential side effects. Moms will gain insights into the importance of hormonal considerations in their treatment plans.

Targeted Therapies

Targeted therapies focus on specific molecules involved in cancer growth, disrupting the pathways that support tumor development. This section explores the concept of targeted therapies, their applications in various cancers, and potential side effects. Moms will learn about the personalized nature of targeted treatments based on the characteristics of their cancer.

Complementary and Integrative Therapies

Complementary and integrative therapies can play a supportive role in cancer treatment. This subsection explores approaches such as acupuncture, massage, and mind-body techniques, emphasizing their potential benefits in managing treatment side effects and improving overall well-being.

Administration Methods

Chemotherapy can be administered in different ways, including:

- Intravenous (IV) Infusions: Direct delivery of drugs into the bloodstream.
- Oral Medications: Pills or liquids taken by mouth.
- Intramuscular or Subcutaneous Injections: Administration into muscle or under the skin.

Moms will learn about the factors influencing the choice of administration method and the implications for treatment.

Treatment Schedule

Chemotherapy is often delivered in cycles, with periods of treatment followed by rest. This subsection explores the typical treatment schedules and the factors influencing the duration and frequency of chemotherapy sessions.

Potential Side Effects

Chemotherapy can lead to a range of side effects, affecting both cancer cells and healthy tissues. Common side effects include:

- Nausea and Vomiting
- Fatigue
- Hair Loss
- Weakened Immune System
- Anemia
- Neuropathy (Nerve Damage)
- Changes in Appetite

Understanding these potential side effects empowers moms to anticipate and manage them effectively.

Managing Side Effects

This section provides practical strategies for managing chemotherapy side effects, including:

- Medications: Prescribed and over-the-counter medications to alleviate symptoms.
- Dietary Adjustments: Tips for managing nausea and maintaining adequate nutrition.
- Emotional Support: Coping strategies and seeking emotional support during treatment.

- Physical Activity: Maintaining physical activity levels to combat fatigue and improve well-being.

Impact on Daily Life

Chemotherapy can have practical implications for daily life. This subsection addresses considerations such as:

- Work and Family Life: Balancing treatment with work and family responsibilities.
- Financial Considerations: Navigating potential financial challenges during treatment.
- Communicating with Healthcare Team: Open communication to address concerns and adjust the treatment plan as needed.

Radiation Therapy

Radiation therapy utilizes high doses of radiation to target and destroy cancer cells or inhibit their growth. It is a localized treatment that aims to minimize damage to healthy surrounding tissues. In this section, moms will gain a comprehensive understanding of radiation therapy, including its goals, the treatment process, potential side effects, and strategies for managing the impact on their well-being.

Goals of Radiation Therapy

Radiation therapy serves various goals, including:

- Curative: Eliminating cancer cells entirely.
- Adjuvant: Destroying remaining cancer cells after surgery or other treatments.
- Palliative: Alleviating symptoms and improving quality of life.

This subsection provides insights into how the goals of radiation therapy are determined based on the type and stage of cancer.

Treatment Planning

Radiation therapy involves meticulous treatment planning to precisely target cancer cells while sparing healthy tissues. Moms will learn about:

- Simulation: Mapping the treatment area using imaging techniques.
- Treatment Fields: Defining the specific areas to receive radiation.
- Dosage Calculation: Determining the appropriate radiation dosage.

- Engage in light exercise, such as walking.
- Communicate fatigue levels with healthcare providers.

Hair Loss

Side Effect:

Chemotherapy can result in hair loss, including eyebrows and eyelashes.

Coping Strategies:

- Consider head coverings, scarves, or wigs.
- Embrace creative ways to express personal style.
- Connect with support groups to share experiences.

Changes in Appetite

Side Effect:

Treatments may alter taste preferences and appetite.

Coping Strategies:

- Experiment with different foods and flavors.
- Opt for small, nutrient-dense meals.
- Discuss nutritional concerns with a dietitian.

Skin Changes

Side Effect:

Radiation therapy and some chemotherapy drugs can cause skin changes.

Coping Strategies:

- Use gentle, fragrance-free skincare products.
- Avoid direct sun exposure to treated areas.
- Communicate changes to healthcare providers promptly.

Emotional Impact

Side Effect:

Cancer treatment can contribute to emotional challenges, including anxiety and depression.

Coping Strategies:

- Seek emotional support from friends, family, or support groups.
- Consider counseling or therapy.
- Engage in activities that bring joy and relaxation.

Neuropathy (Nerve Damage)

Side Effect:

Certain chemotherapy drugs may cause tingling or numbness in the hands and feet.

Coping Strategies:

- Report symptoms promptly to healthcare providers.
- Opt for gentle exercises like walking.
- Use assistive devices if needed.

Managing Treatment-Related Challenges

Coping Strategies:

- Maintain open communication with healthcare providers about side effects.
- Attend support groups to share experiences and coping strategies.
- Prioritize self-care, including adequate rest and relaxation.

Communicating with Healthcare Providers

Coping Strategies:

- Report any unusual or severe side effects promptly.
- Ask questions about potential side effects before starting treatment.
- Collaborate with healthcare providers to adjust the treatment plan if needed.

Chapter 3: Emotional Impact on Moms

A cancer diagnosis and the subsequent journey through treatment can have profound emotional effects on moms. Understanding and addressing these emotional challenges is a crucial aspect of holistic cancer care. In this section, we explore the emotional impact of cancer on moms and provide strategies for coping with the complex range of feelings that may arise.

Initial Reactions and Shock

Emotional Impact:

Receiving a cancer diagnosis can evoke shock, disbelief, fear, and a range of intense emotions.

Coping Strategies:

- Allow time for emotional processing.
- Seek support from loved ones.
- Consider talking to a mental health professional.

Anxiety and Uncertainty

Emotional Impact:

Anxiety may arise from uncertainty about the future, treatment outcomes, and the impact on family life.

Coping Strategies:

- Practice mindfulness and relaxation techniques.
- Engage in open communication with healthcare providers.
- Establish a support network for emotional reassurance.

Depression and Sadness

Emotional Impact:

The challenges of cancer may lead to feelings of sadness, grief, and depression.

Coping Strategies:

- Reach out for professional counseling or therapy.
- Engage in activities that bring joy and relaxation.
- Prioritize self-care and emotional well-being.

Fear of the Unknown

Emotional Impact:

Uncertainty about treatment outcomes, potential changes in appearance, and the impact on daily life can lead to fear.

Coping Strategies:

- Educate oneself about the treatment process.
- Share fears and concerns with healthcare providers.
- Connect with others who have experienced similar situations.

Impact on Relationships

Emotional Impact:

Cancer can strain relationships due to changing roles, emotional stress, and communication challenges.

Coping Strategies:

- Foster open communication with family members.
- Seek couples or family counseling if needed.
- Share feelings and concerns to maintain connection.

Guilt and Self-blame

Emotional Impact:

Moms may experience guilt or self-blame, questioning if they could have prevented the cancer.

Coping Strategies:

- Acknowledge that cancer is not one's fault.
- Seek support from loved ones and professionals.
- Focus on self-compassion and acceptance.

Coping with Treatment Side Effects

Emotional Impact:

Dealing with physical changes, such as hair loss or fatigue, can impact self-esteem and body image.

Coping Strategies:

- Embrace support from loved ones.
- Connect with others who have experienced similar side effects.
- Consider support groups or counseling to address body image concerns.

Celebrating Small Victories

Emotional Impact:

Acknowledging and celebrating small victories in the treatment journey can bring a sense of accomplishment.

Coping Strategies:

- Recognize and celebrate milestones.
- Establish personal goals and rewards.
- Share successes with supportive friends and family.

Advocating for Emotional Well-being

Coping Strategies:

- Communicate emotional needs with healthcare providers.
- Seek referrals to mental health professionals.
- Engage in activities that promote emotional well-being.

Coping with the Initial Diagnosis

The moment of receiving a cancer diagnosis can be overwhelming and emotionally charged. Coping with the initial diagnosis is a critical phase that sets the tone for the entire cancer journey. In this section, moms will find guidance on navigating the complex emotions and practical steps to cope with the initial impact of a cancer diagnosis.

Allow Yourself to Feel

Coping Strategies:

- Acknowledge Emotions: Understand that a range of emotions, including shock, fear, and sadness, is natural.
- Express Feelings: Share your emotions with trusted friends, family, or a mental health professional.
- Give Yourself Time: Allow yourself the time needed to process and come to terms with the diagnosis.

Seek Information and Understanding

Coping Strategies:

- Ask Questions: Don't hesitate to ask your healthcare team about the diagnosis, treatment options, and what to expect.
- Educate Yourself: Gather information from reputable sources to understand the type and stage of cancer.
- Take Notes: Bring a notebook to appointments to jot down information and questions.

Build a Support Network

Coping Strategies:

- Share with Loved Ones: Inform close friends and family about the diagnosis for emotional support.
- Join Support Groups: Connect with others who have experienced similar diagnoses to share experiences and advice.
- Lean on Professionals: Seek guidance from social workers or counselors provided by the healthcare team.

Prioritize Self-Care

Coping Strategies:

- Rest and Recharge: Ensure you get adequate rest and prioritize self-care.
- Healthy Habits: Maintain a balanced diet and engage in gentle exercises, as allowed by your healthcare team.
- Mindfulness Practices: Consider practices such as meditation or yoga for stress reduction.

Make Informed Decisions

Coping Strategies:

- Collaborate with Healthcare Team: Work closely with your healthcare team to understand treatment options and make informed decisions.
- Seek Second Opinions: Don't hesitate to seek a second opinion to ensure confidence in the proposed treatment plan.
- Consider Treatment Preferences: Discuss treatment preferences, potential side effects, and long-term implications with your healthcare team.

Address Practical Concerns

Coping Strategies:

- Financial Planning: Consider the potential impact of treatment on finances and explore resources for financial support.
- Workplace Communication: Communicate with your employer about your situation and explore options for managing work responsibilities.
- Legal and Administrative Tasks: Address legal and administrative tasks promptly, such as updating wills and organizing important documents.

Embrace Emotional Support

Coping Strategies:

- Therapeutic Interventions: Consider counseling or therapy to address emotional challenges.
- Express Your Needs: Clearly communicate your emotional needs to friends, family, and your healthcare team.
- Engage in Activities You Enjoy: Continue participating in activities that bring joy and fulfillment.

Set Realistic Expectations

Coping Strategies:

- Accept Uncertainty: Understand that the cancer journey may involve uncertainty, and setting realistic expectations can reduce anxiety.
- Celebrate Small Victories: Acknowledge and celebrate small milestones and positive moments during treatment.

Communicating with Family and Children

Sharing a cancer diagnosis with family, especially children, is a delicate and important aspect of the cancer journey. Effective communication can foster understanding, provide emotional support, and help everyone involved navigate the challenges ahead. In this section, we explore strategies for communicating the diagnosis with family members, including children, in a compassionate and supportive manner.

Timing and Setting

Communication Strategies:

- Choose a Calm Setting: Find a quiet and comfortable space for the conversation, minimizing distractions.
- Timing is Key: Pick a time when everyone can be present and focus on the discussion.
- Consider Individual Preferences: Some family members may prefer immediate discussions, while others may need time to process the news.

Be Honest and Direct

Communication Strategies:

- Use Clear Language: Explain the diagnosis using language that is age-appropriate and understandable.
- Avoid Ambiguity: Be honest about the situation without creating unnecessary confusion or false hope.
- Address Fears and Concerns: Encourage questions and address concerns openly.

Provide Age-Appropriate Information for Children

Communication Strategies:

- Use Simple Language: Tailor explanations to the child's age, using simple and concrete terms.
- Focus on Reassurance: Emphasize that the illness is not the child's fault, and that there are caregivers and healthcare professionals to help.
- Offer Reassurance of Love: Ensure the child understands that they are loved and will be supported throughout the process.

Encourage Expressing Emotions

Communication Strategies:

- Create an Open Environment: Establish an atmosphere where family members, including children, feel comfortable expressing their emotions.
- Validate Feelings: Acknowledge and validate the diverse emotions family members may be experiencing.
- Model Healthy Expression: Demonstrate healthy ways of coping with emotions, encouraging open communication.

Answer Questions Honestly

Communication Strategies:

- Be Prepared: Anticipate potential questions and be prepared to answer them honestly.
- Acknowledge Limits: If there are uncertainties, communicate that some aspects are not fully known yet.
- Reassure Support: Emphasize that there will be ongoing communication and support throughout the journey.

Involve Healthcare Professionals

Communication Strategies:

- Facilitate Healthcare Provider Discussions: Allow space for the involvement of healthcare professionals in discussions, especially for answering specific medical questions.
- Arrange Family Meetings: Consider arranging meetings with healthcare providers to discuss the diagnosis and treatment plan together as a family.

Addressing Sibling Dynamics

Communication Strategies:

- Equal Attention: Ensure each child receives equal attention and information based on their age and understanding.
- Foster Sibling Support: Encourage siblings to support each other and express their feelings.
- Be Mindful of Age Differences: Tailor communication to the developmental stage of each child.

Offer Reassurance and Stability

Communication Strategies:

- Highlight Support Systems: Emphasize the presence of a strong support system, including family, friends, and healthcare professionals.
- Maintain Routines: Whenever possible, maintain normal routines to provide a sense of stability for children and family members.
- Reassure Love and Commitment: Reiterate the enduring love and commitment within the family despite the challenges.

Seek Professional Guidance if Needed

Communication Strategies:

- Family Counseling: Consider family counseling to facilitate open communication and provide a safe space for everyone to express their feelings.
- Child Life Specialists: Involve child life specialists in the hospital setting to support children through age-appropriate interventions.

Managing Emotional Well-being

Emotional well-being is a vital aspect of navigating the challenges of a cancer journey. Fostering resilience, seeking support, and incorporating self-care practices are essential components of maintaining emotional well-being. In this section, moms will find strategies and insights to manage their emotional health throughout the various stages of the cancer experience.

Prioritize Self-Care

Strategies:

- Rest and Sleep: Ensure adequate rest and prioritize quality sleep for physical and emotional rejuvenation.
- Nutrition: Maintain a balanced diet to support overall well-being.
- Gentle Exercise: Engage in gentle exercises, as approved by healthcare professionals, to boost mood and reduce stress.
- Mindfulness Practices: Incorporate mindfulness, meditation, or deep-breathing exercises to promote relaxation.

Seek Emotional Support

Strategies:

- Build a Support Network: Surround yourself with understanding friends, family, and support groups who can provide emotional support.
- Professional Counseling: Consider individual or group counseling to address emotional challenges and coping strategies.
- Online Communities: Explore online communities and forums where individuals share experiences and provide mutual support.

Communicate Openly

Strategies:

- Express Feelings: Share your thoughts and feelings with trusted friends, family, or a mental health professional.
- Open Dialogue: Encourage open communication within the family about emotional well-being and concerns.
- Journaling: Consider keeping a journal to express thoughts and emotions privately.

Set Realistic Expectations

Strategies:

- Accept Uncertainty: Acknowledge that the cancer journey may involve uncertainties, and setting realistic expectations can reduce anxiety.
- Celebrate Small Victories: Acknowledge and celebrate small milestones and positive moments during the treatment process.
- Adjust Goals: Be flexible in adjusting personal and professional goals based on energy levels and priorities.

Engage in Enjoyable Activities

Strategies:

- Hobbies and Interests: Continue pursuing hobbies and interests that bring joy and a sense of accomplishment.
- Cultural and Recreational Activities: Attend cultural events, concerts, or recreational activities that contribute to a positive mindset.

- Quality Time with Loved Ones: Spend quality time with loved ones in activities that foster connection and enjoyment.

Manage Stress Effectively

Strategies:

- Stress-Reduction Techniques: Practice stress-reduction techniques such as yoga, meditation, or guided imagery.
- Time Management: Prioritize tasks and manage time effectively to reduce feelings of overwhelm.
- Set Boundaries: Establish and communicate clear boundaries to manage external stressors.

Address Grief and Loss

Strategies:

- Grief Processing: Allow time and space to grieve losses, whether related to health, lifestyle, or expectations.
- Professional Guidance: Seek support from grief counselors or support groups to navigate feelings of loss.
- Memorialization: Consider creating meaningful rituals or memorials to honor what has been lost.

Embrace Positive Thinking

Strategies:

- Cultivate Gratitude: Practice gratitude by acknowledging and appreciating positive aspects of life.
- Positive Affirmations: Incorporate positive affirmations into daily routines to foster a positive mindset.
- Visualizations: Use visualization techniques to imagine positive outcomes and a hopeful future.

Advocacy for Mental Health

Strategies:

- Communicate Needs: Clearly communicate emotional needs with healthcare providers to ensure comprehensive care.

- Participate in Decision-Making: Actively participate in treatment decisions to align with personal preferences and well-being.
- Seek Professional Input: Consult with mental health professionals as needed to address specific emotional concerns.

Chapter 4: Practical Matters

Addressing practical matters during a cancer journey is essential for minimizing stress and ensuring a smooth and well-supported experience. This section provides guidance on managing practical aspects related to finances, work, legal considerations, and other logistical concerns that may arise.

Financial Planning and Resources

Strategies:

- Review Finances: Assess current financial situations, including income, savings, and expenses.
- Explore Insurance Coverage: Understand health insurance coverage and explore available financial assistance programs.
- Create a Budget: Develop a budget that accounts for medical costs, daily expenses, and potential changes in income.
- Seek Financial Assistance: Explore financial assistance programs offered by cancer organizations, hospitals, or government agencies.

Workplace Communication and Support

Strategies:

- Notify Employers: Communicate with employers about the diagnosis, treatment plan, and potential changes to work schedules.
- Explore Flexible Work Arrangements: Discuss flexible work options, such as remote work or adjusted hours, to accommodate treatment needs.
- Know Employment Rights: Understand employment rights and protections provided by laws such as the Family and Medical Leave Act (FMLA).

Legal and Administrative Tasks

Strategies:

- Update Legal Documents: Review and update legal documents, including wills, powers of attorney, and healthcare directives.
- Organize Important Documents: Gather and organize essential documents, such as medical records, insurance policies, and financial statements.
- Consider Guardianship for Children: Address considerations related to guardianship for children, if applicable.
- Seek Legal Advice: Consult with legal professionals for guidance on specific legal matters and considerations.

Transportation and Logistics

Strategies:

- Coordinate Transportation: Plan for transportation to and from medical appointments, considering potential challenges during treatment.
- Explore Community Resources: Investigate available community resources that may provide transportation assistance.
- Organize Support Networks: Establish a network of friends and family who can assist with transportation needs.

Child and Family Care

Strategies:

- Arrange Child Care: Plan for childcare during medical appointments, treatments, and recovery periods.
- Coordinate Family Support: Communicate with extended family members or friends who can provide additional support for children and family members.
- Discuss Family Responsibilities: Have open discussions with family members about potential shifts in responsibilities and roles.

Home Environment and Adaptations

Strategies:

- Create a Comfortable Home Environment: Ensure the home environment is comfortable and supportive during treatment and recovery.
- Consider Home Adaptations: Evaluate potential home adaptations, such as handrails or ramps, to enhance safety.
- Discuss Needs with Healthcare Providers: Communicate home-related needs with healthcare providers for personalized advice.

Care Coordination and Medical Records

Strategies:

- Centralize Medical Records: Maintain a centralized system for organizing and accessing medical records.
- Coordinate Care Plans: Facilitate communication between healthcare providers to ensure a cohesive and coordinated care plan.
- Designate a Point of Contact: Designate a point of contact for coordinating appointments and communicating with the healthcare team.

Community Support and Resources

Strategies:

- Tap into Local Resources: Explore local cancer support organizations, community services, and resources that can provide practical assistance.
- Connect with Support Groups: Join support groups where members can share practical tips and insights.
- Utilize Online Platforms: Leverage online platforms and resources that offer guidance on practical matters related to cancer.

Navigating Healthcare Systems

Effectively navigating healthcare systems is crucial for receiving optimal care and support during a cancer journey. This section provides strategies to empower moms in understanding, accessing, and collaborating with healthcare providers to ensure comprehensive and personalized care.

Establishing Open Communication with Healthcare Providers

Strategies:

- Ask Questions: Don't hesitate to ask questions about the diagnosis, treatment options, and potential side effects.
- Create a List of Questions: Prepare a list of questions before appointments to ensure all concerns are addressed.
- Seek Second Opinions: If needed, seek second opinions to explore various perspectives on the diagnosis and treatment plan.

Building a Healthcare Team

Strategies:

- Identify Key Healthcare Professionals: Recognize the roles of various healthcare professionals, including oncologists, nurses, social workers, and specialists.
- Collaborate with Primary Care Physicians: Keep primary care physicians informed and involved in the overall healthcare plan.
- Utilize Support Services: Take advantage of support services offered by hospitals, such as counseling, nutrition services, and rehabilitation.

Understanding Treatment Plans and Options

Strategies:

- Request a Clear Treatment Plan: Ensure that treatment plans are clearly explained, outlining the goals, timeline, and potential side effects.
- Discuss Alternative Treatments: Explore alternative or complementary therapies, ensuring they align with the overall treatment plan.
- Participate in Decision-Making: Actively participate in decisions about treatment options, expressing personal preferences and values.

Managing Appointments and Scheduling

Strategies:

- Organize Appointments: Keep track of appointments using a calendar or scheduling tool to avoid missed or overlapping dates.
- Coordinate Multiple Providers: If seeing multiple healthcare providers, ensure coordination to avoid conflicts in scheduling.
- Communicate Changes Promptly: Inform healthcare providers promptly about any changes in the schedule or health status.

Accessing Medical Records and Information

Strategies:

- Centralized Medical Records: Maintain a centralized location for storing and organizing medical records for easy access.
- Request Copies of Records: Request copies of medical records, test results, and imaging studies for personal reference.
- Utilize Online Portals: Take advantage of online patient portals offered by healthcare providers for convenient access to medical information.

Advocating for Comprehensive Care

Strategies:

- Express Concerns and Preferences: Communicate openly with healthcare providers about personal concerns, preferences, and goals for care.
- Request Multidisciplinary Meetings: Advocate for multidisciplinary meetings where different specialists collaborate to optimize care.
- Seek Referrals When Needed: Request referrals to specialists or support services when necessary for comprehensive care.

Understanding Insurance Coverage and Billing

Strategies:

- Review Insurance Policies: Understand insurance coverage, including copayments, deductibles, and restrictions.
- Clarify Billing Questions: If unsure about a bill or charges, contact the billing department promptly for clarification.
- Explore Financial Assistance: Inquire about financial assistance programs or support offered by hospitals and cancer organizations.

Advocacy for Personalized Care

Strategies:

- Voice Preferences and Concerns: Advocate for personalized care that aligns with individual preferences and concerns.
- Discuss Quality of Life Priorities: Share priorities related to quality of life, including family, work, and personal goals.
- Be an Active Participant: Actively participate in decisions about care and treatment options, contributing to the development of a personalized care plan.

Financial Considerations and Resources

Managing the financial aspects of a cancer journey is crucial for minimizing stress and ensuring access to necessary resources. This section provides guidance on navigating financial considerations, exploring available resources, and seeking assistance to alleviate potential financial burdens.

Assessing Financial Impact

Strategies:

- Review Insurance Coverage: Understand the details of health insurance coverage, including deductibles, copayments, and coverage limitations.
- Evaluate Out-of-Pocket Costs: Anticipate and budget for out-of-pocket costs associated with medical treatments, medications, and supportive care.
- Assess Income Changes: Consider potential changes in income due to work disruptions or adjustments.

Exploring Financial Assistance Programs

Strategies:

- Inquire About Hospital Assistance: Contact the financial assistance or billing department of the treating hospital to inquire about available programs.
- Research Nonprofit Organizations: Explore nonprofit organizations dedicated to supporting individuals with cancer, such as CancerCare, Patient Advocate Foundation, and local cancer charities.
- Check Government Assistance Programs: Investigate government assistance programs that provide financial support for medical expenses.

Creating a Budget and Financial Plan

Strategies:

- Develop a Detailed Budget: Create a detailed budget that outlines income, expenses, and anticipated medical costs.
- Prioritize Essential Expenses: Identify and prioritize essential expenses, ensuring that medical and treatment costs are adequately accounted for.
- Seek Financial Counseling: Consider seeking financial counseling or advice from professionals to develop a comprehensive financial plan.

Negotiating Medical Bills

Strategies:

- Review and Understand Bills: Carefully review medical bills to ensure accuracy and understanding of charges.

- Communicate with Providers: Reach out to healthcare providers to discuss and negotiate payment plans, discounts, or financial assistance.
- Request Itemized Statements: Request itemized statements to gain a clear understanding of billed charges.

Utilizing Health Savings Accounts (HSAs) and Flexible Spending Accounts (FSAs)

Strategies:

- Maximize Contributions: If applicable, maximize contributions to HSAs and FSAs to cover eligible medical expenses.
- Understand Eligible Expenses: Familiarize yourself with the types of medical expenses covered by HSAs and FSAs.
- Plan for Future Costs: Use these accounts strategically to plan for future medical costs, including copayments and deductibles.

Seeking Legal and Financial Advice

Strategies:

- Consult with Financial Advisors: Seek advice from financial advisors to explore investment options, savings strategies, and potential impacts on long-term financial goals.
- Legal Consultation: Consider consulting with legal professionals to address estate planning, wills, and other legal considerations.
- Explore Social Security Disability Benefits: If applicable, explore the possibility of applying for Social Security Disability benefits.

Exploring Community Resources

Strategies:

- Connect with Local Charities: Reach out to local charities and community organizations that may offer financial assistance or support services.
- Explore Transportation Assistance: Investigate transportation assistance programs that can help with the costs of commuting to medical appointments.
- Look for Housing Support: If applicable, explore housing support or temporary lodging options for those undergoing treatment away from home.

Communicating with Employers

Strategies:

- Understand Employment Benefits: Familiarize yourself with employment benefits, including sick leave, vacation time, and short-term disability options.
- Discuss Work Arrangements: Engage in open communication with employers about potential work adjustments, flexible schedules, or remote work options.
- Inquire About Employee Assistance Programs (EAPs): Check if your employer offers Employee Assistance Programs that provide counseling and support services.

Managing Debt and Credit

Strategies:

- Communicate with Creditors: If facing financial challenges, communicate with creditors to discuss potential hardship programs or arrangements.
- Prioritize Debt Repayment: Establish priorities for debt repayment, focusing on essential expenses and medical bills.
- Monitor Credit Reports: Regularly monitor credit reports to ensure accuracy and address any discrepancies.

Seeking Pro Bono Legal Services

Strategies:

- Contact Legal Aid Organizations: Explore pro bono legal services offered by legal aid organizations or law firms that provide support to individuals facing financial hardship.
- Check with Cancer Support Organizations: Some cancer support organizations may have partnerships with legal professionals offering pro bono services.

Balancing Work and Cancer

Juggling the responsibilities of work while undergoing cancer treatment can be challenging, but with careful planning and open communication, it is possible to strike a balance. This section offers strategies for moms navigating the delicate balance between their professional and health-related commitments during a cancer journey.

Open Communication with Employers

Strategies:

- Notify Employers Early: Inform employers about the cancer diagnosis as early as possible, providing sufficient details about treatment plans and potential work adjustments.
- Discuss Treatment Schedule: Have open discussions about the treatment schedule, including appointments and potential time off.
- Explore Flexible Work Arrangements: Work with employers to explore flexible work arrangements, such as part-time schedules, remote work, or adjusted hours.

Understanding Employment Rights

Strategies:

- Know Legal Protections: Understand employment rights and legal protections provided by laws such as the Family and Medical Leave Act (FMLA) or the Americans with Disabilities Act (ADA).
- Review Company Policies: Familiarize yourself with your company's policies related to medical leave, disability accommodations, and benefits during illness.
- Consult with Human Resources: Seek guidance from human resources to understand available options and support services.

Prioritizing Self-Care and Health

Strategies:

- Communicate Health Needs: Clearly communicate health needs and limitations to employers, emphasizing the importance of prioritizing self-care during treatment.
- Set Realistic Expectations: Establish realistic expectations for work responsibilities, workload, and deadlines during the treatment period.
- Advocate for Breaks: Advocate for breaks and rest periods as needed, especially during days of treatment or when experiencing fatigue.

Planning for Absences and Leave

Strategies:

- Coordinate Leave Periods: Coordinate planned absences, such as medical appointments and treatment days, with supervisors and colleagues.

- Explore Paid Time Off (PTO): Utilize accrued paid time off for medical appointments, treatment days, or recovery periods.
- Understand Leave Policies: Understand company policies regarding medical leave, disability leave, and other forms of time off.

*Collaborating with Co-workers and Supervisors**

Strategies:

- Maintain Open Communication: Keep lines of communication open with co-workers and supervisors, providing updates on treatment progress and potential changes in work arrangements.
- Delegate Tasks: Delegate tasks or responsibilities to colleagues during periods of increased medical appointments or treatment intensity.
- Build a Supportive Network: Build a supportive network at work, fostering an environment where colleagues can offer assistance and understanding.

Exploring Workplace Support Services

Strategies:

- Employee Assistance Programs (EAPs): Utilize Employee Assistance Programs if available, which may offer counseling, mental health support, and resources for managing work-related stress.
- Workplace Accommodations: Discuss potential workplace accommodations, such as ergonomic adjustments, flexible schedules, or modified duties to accommodate health needs.
- Counseling Services: Seek counseling services or support groups facilitated by the workplace or external organizations to address the emotional impact of cancer.

Time Management and Productivity Strategies

Strategies:

- Prioritize Tasks: Prioritize tasks and focus on high-priority assignments while managing energy levels during treatment.
- Use Time Management Tools: Utilize time management tools, calendars, and productivity apps to stay organized and on top of work commitments.
- Communicate Work Capacity: Communicate openly with supervisors and colleagues about work capacity, ensuring realistic expectations are set.

Exploring Remote Work Options

Strategies:

- Discuss Remote Work: If feasible, discuss the possibility of remote work with employers, especially during periods of treatment or when managing side effects.
- Establish Remote Work Guidelines: Establish clear guidelines for remote work, including communication channels, expectations, and regular check-ins.
- Utilize Technology: Leverage technology tools and platforms that facilitate remote collaboration and communication with the team.

Coping with Work-Related Stress and Emotions

Strategies:

- Seek Emotional Support: Seek emotional support from colleagues, friends, or support groups to cope with work-related stress and emotions.
- Set Boundaries: Establish clear boundaries between work and personal life, ensuring time for self-care and relaxation.
- Consider Professional Counseling: Consider professional counseling or therapy to address work-related stress and emotional challenges.

Planning for Return to Work

Strategies:

- Gradual Return: Plan for a gradual return to work, starting with reduced hours or modified duties if needed.
- Discuss Accommodations: Discuss any necessary accommodations with employers and supervisors to ensure a smooth transition back to full-time work.
- Communicate Changes: Communicate openly about any changes in work capacity or needs that arise during the return-to-work period.

Support Systems

Building and maintaining a strong support system is crucial for moms facing a cancer journey. Having a network of understanding and caring individuals can provide emotional, practical, and spiritual support. This section explores strategies for cultivating and utilizing support systems during challenging times.

Identifying Key Supportive Individuals

Strategies:

- Family and Friends: Strengthen connections with close family members and friends who can offer emotional support, assistance with daily tasks, and companionship.
- Healthcare Team: Build a positive and communicative relationship with healthcare professionals, including oncologists, nurses, and support staff.
- Community and Support Groups: Connect with local cancer support groups, online communities, and organizations that provide a sense of belonging and shared experiences.

Open Communication within the Family

Strategies:

- Family Meetings: Schedule family meetings to discuss the cancer journey, share updates, and address concerns together.
- Encourage Expressiveness: Foster an environment where family members feel comfortable expressing their emotions and concerns.
- Clarify Roles and Responsibilities: Clearly define roles and responsibilities within the family, acknowledging the contributions of each member.

Building a Supportive Friend Network

Strategies:

- Selective Disclosure: Choose trusted friends to share the cancer diagnosis and treatment journey, ensuring a supportive and understanding network.
- Coordinate Help: Organize friends into a support team that can assist with practical tasks, emotional support, or childcare.
- Regular Check-Ins: Establish regular check-ins with friends to maintain ongoing communication and receive consistent support.

Utilizing Professional Support Services

Strategies:

- Therapists and Counselors: Seek the services of therapists or counselors who specialize in cancer-related emotional support for both individuals and families.
- Social Workers: Engage with social workers available through healthcare facilities for assistance with practical and emotional aspects of the cancer journey.

- Child Life Specialists: If applicable, involve child life specialists to support children through age-appropriate interventions.

Exploring Spiritual and Faith-Based Support*

Strategies:

- Spiritual Leaders: Connect with spiritual leaders, such as clergy or chaplains, for emotional and spiritual guidance.
- Faith Communities: Engage with faith communities and support groups that align with personal spiritual beliefs.
- Participate in Spiritual Practices: Incorporate personal spiritual practices, such as prayer or meditation, to find strength and comfort.

Engaging with Supportive Organizations

Strategies:

- Cancer Support Organizations: Seek assistance and resources from cancer support organizations that offer services, support groups, and educational materials.
- Local Community Services: Explore local community services, such as meal assistance programs, transportation services, and financial aid provided by charitable organizations.
- Online Platforms: Utilize online platforms and forums where individuals share experiences and offer support.

Maintaining Healthy Relationships

Strategies:

- Open Communication with Partners: Foster open communication with partners, ensuring shared decision-making and mutual understanding.
- Quality Time with Children: Spend quality time with children, engaging in age-appropriate activities and addressing their emotional needs.
- Balancing Independence: Encourage family members to balance independence with interdependence, allowing for personal growth and support.

Self-Care and Personal Support*

Strategies:

- Prioritizing Self-Care: Emphasize the importance of self-care for both physical and emotional well-being.
- Seeking Individual Counseling: Consider individual counseling or therapy to address personal challenges and emotions.
- Connecting with Supportive Individuals: Identify and connect with individuals who offer personal support, understanding, and companionship.

Communication Guidelines with Support Systems

Strategies:

- Expressing Needs Clearly: Clearly communicate personal needs and preferences to support individuals, fostering effective and meaningful assistance.
- Setting Boundaries: Establish clear boundaries to ensure a balance between receiving support and maintaining personal space.
- Regular Updates: Provide regular updates to support systems about the treatment process, progress, and any changes in needs.

Embracing Community and Volunteer Support

Strategies:

- Engaging with Community Events: Participate in community events, fundraisers, or support walks to connect with others facing similar challenges.
- Volunteer Assistance: If available, consider accepting volunteer assistance for tasks such as meal preparation, transportation, or household chores.
- Local Community Resources: Explore local community resources that offer assistance and support to families affected by cancer.

Building a Support Network

Building a strong support network is essential for moms navigating a cancer journey. A well-rounded network can provide emotional, practical, and social support during challenging times. This section outlines strategies for moms to actively build and strengthen their support networks.

Identifying Key Individuals

Strategies:

- Family Members: Strengthen connections with immediate family members, such as a spouse, children, parents, and siblings.

- Close Friends: Reach out to close friends who have shown understanding, empathy, and a willingness to provide support.
- Extended Family: Connect with extended family members who can offer additional support and assistance.
- Neighbors and Community: Build relationships with neighbors and community members who may provide practical assistance and companionship.

Communicating Openly

Strategies:

- Share Personal Story: Openly share the cancer diagnosis, treatment plan, and emotional experiences with selected individuals in the support network.
- Express Needs Clearly: Clearly communicate specific needs, whether they are emotional support, practical assistance, or companionship.
- Encourage Open Dialogue: Foster an environment where individuals feel comfortable expressing their own feelings and concerns.

Building a Care Team

Strategies:

- Healthcare Professionals: Establish open communication and collaboration with healthcare professionals, including oncologists, nurses, and social workers.
- Therapists and Counselors: Engage with therapists or counselors who specialize in cancer-related emotional support for both individuals and families.
- Support Groups: Join local or online cancer support groups where moms can connect with others facing similar challenges.

Engaging with Social and Community Networks

Strategies:

- Community Organizations: Connect with local cancer support organizations, community centers, and charities that offer assistance, resources, and events.
- Religious or Spiritual Communities: Engage with religious or spiritual communities that provide emotional and spiritual support.
- Participate in Community Events: Attend community events, workshops, or gatherings that facilitate connections with supportive individuals.

Seeking Professional Support Services

Strategies:

- Social Workers: Utilize the services of social workers available through healthcare facilities to address practical and emotional aspects of the cancer journey.
- Child Life Specialists: If applicable, involve child life specialists to support children through age-appropriate interventions.
- Counselors: Seek the services of counselors or therapists to address emotional challenges and provide coping strategies.

Expanding Social Circles

Strategies:

- Meetup Groups: Explore local meetup groups focused on shared interests, hobbies, or activities to expand social circles.
- Parenting Groups: Connect with parenting groups or playdate communities where moms can find companionship and shared experiences.
- Online Platforms: Utilize online platforms and forums to connect with individuals who share similar challenges or interests.

Incorporating Supportive Professionals

Strategies:

- Legal and Financial Advisors: Engage with legal and financial professionals who can provide guidance on legal matters, financial planning, and resources.
- Health Advocates: Consider involving health advocates or patient navigators who can assist in coordinating care, addressing insurance issues, and providing information.
- Educational Professionals: Communicate with school administrators, teachers, and counselors to ensure support for children's educational needs during the cancer journey.

Participating in Supportive Activities

Strategies:

- Exercise and Wellness Classes: Join exercise or wellness classes that offer physical and mental health benefits while providing opportunities to meet supportive individuals.
- Art or Creative Workshops: Explore art or creative workshops that can serve as therapeutic outlets and foster connections with like-minded individuals.

- Volunteer Opportunities: Consider engaging in volunteer activities, where moms can connect with others while contributing to meaningful causes.

Fostering Mutual Support

Strategies:

- Reciprocal Relationships: Encourage mutual support by offering assistance or companionship to others within the support network.
- Shared Responsibilities: Collaborate with family members and friends to share responsibilities, reducing the burden on any single individual.
- Celebrate Achievements: Acknowledge and celebrate achievements, milestones, and positive moments within the support network.

Embracing Cultural or Diversity-Based Communities

Strategies:

- Cultural or Ethnic Groups: Connect with cultural or ethnic communities that provide understanding and support, addressing unique cultural needs.
- Multicultural Events: Attend multicultural events and activities to build connections with individuals from diverse backgrounds.

Joining Support Groups

Joining support groups can provide valuable emotional, informational, and practical assistance for moms navigating a cancer journey. These groups offer a sense of community, shared experiences, and a supportive environment. This section outlines strategies for moms to effectively join and benefit from support groups.

Researching Local and Online Support Groups

Strategies:

- Local Cancer Centers: Inquire with local cancer treatment centers or hospitals about available support groups for individuals and families.
- Online Platforms: Explore online platforms and websites that host virtual support groups, allowing for participation from the comfort of home.

- Community Organizations: Connect with community organizations, charities, or non-profits that may facilitate support groups for cancer patients and their families.

Choosing the Right Support Group

Strategies:

- Disease-Specific Groups: Consider joining support groups that focus on the specific type of cancer being addressed, providing targeted information and shared experiences.
- Stage-Specific Groups: Look for groups tailored to the stage of the cancer journey, such as those for individuals in treatment, survivors, or those facing advanced stages.
- Parenting or Mom-Focused Groups: Seek out support groups specifically designed for mothers navigating a cancer journey, addressing the unique challenges and concerns they may face.

Attending In-Person or Virtual Meetings

Strategies:

- Check Meeting Schedules: Review the meeting schedules of local or online support groups and choose those that align with personal availability.
- Prepare for Virtual Meetings: If attending virtual meetings, familiarize yourself with the online platform and ensure a quiet and comfortable space for participation.
- Participate Actively: Engage actively in discussions, share personal experiences, and ask questions during group meetings to make the most of the support network.

Inquiring About Group Dynamics and Facilitation

Strategies:

- Contact Group Facilitators: Reach out to the facilitators or organizers of support groups to inquire about group dynamics, format, and any specific guidelines.
- Attend a Trial Session: Consider attending a trial session to get a feel for the group dynamics and determine if it aligns with personal preferences and needs.
- Feedback and Suggestions: Provide feedback and suggestions to group facilitators to enhance the overall experience for participants.

Building Connections with Group Members

Strategies:

- Introduce Yourself: Take the opportunity to introduce yourself during group meetings, sharing a brief overview of your situation and concerns.
- Initiate One-on-One Conversations: Reach out to individuals within the group for one-on-one conversations to deepen connections and exchange support.
- Be Open to Connecting: Be open to connecting with individuals who may have different experiences, as diverse perspectives can enrich the support network.

Contributing to Group Discussions

Strategies:

- Share Personal Experiences: Share your own experiences, challenges, and successes during group discussions to contribute to the collective knowledge and understanding.
- Ask Questions: Ask questions to gain insights from others who may have faced similar situations or have valuable information.
- Offer Support to Others: Extend support and encouragement to fellow group members, fostering a sense of camaraderie within the community.

Balancing Listening and Sharing

Strategies:

- Practice Active Listening: Engage in active listening during group discussions, allowing others to share their experiences without interruption.
- Express Personal Needs: When appropriate, express your own needs and concerns, balancing the sharing of personal experiences with receptivity to others.
- Respect Privacy: Respect the privacy of others within the group and avoid pressuring individuals to share more than they are comfortable with.

Leveraging Online Resources

Strategies:

- Explore Online Forums: Apart from scheduled meetings, explore online forums or discussion boards associated with support groups for continuous communication and information exchange.
- Utilize Group Resources: Take advantage of resources provided by the support group, such as educational materials, articles, and recommended readings.
- Stay Informed: Regularly check group websites or online platforms for updates, announcements, and additional resources.

Managing Expectations

Strategies:

- Be Realistic: Set realistic expectations about the level of involvement and support that can be gained from the group.
- Evaluate Personal Comfort: Continuously evaluate personal comfort and satisfaction within the group, considering whether adjustments or changes are needed.
- Explore Multiple Groups: If available, explore participation in multiple groups to find the one that best aligns with personal preferences and needs.

Seeking Professional Guidance if Needed

Strategies:

- Therapeutic Support: If facing emotional challenges beyond what the support group provides, consider seeking therapeutic support from individual counseling or therapy.
- Consult Healthcare Professionals: Consult with healthcare professionals, such as social workers or psychologists, for guidance on additional support resources and coping strategies.
- Be Open to Varied Support: Recognize that support can come from various sources, including support groups, friends, family, and professionals, and be open to leveraging multiple avenues.

Communicating with Healthcare Professionals

Effective communication with healthcare professionals is crucial for moms navigating a cancer journey. Clear and open communication ensures that all aspects of the diagnosis, treatment, and overall care are well understood. This section provides strategies for moms to communicate effectively with their healthcare team.

Establishing Open Communication Channels

Strategies:

- Create a Communication Plan: Develop a communication plan that outlines how and when to communicate with healthcare professionals, including scheduled appointments, emails, or phone calls.
- Understand Preferred Communication Methods: Inquire about healthcare providers' preferred communication methods, whether it's through the patient portal, phone calls, or in-person meetings.

- Identify Key Contacts: Recognize key contacts within the healthcare team, such as the primary oncologist, nurse, and social worker, to facilitate smoother communication.

Asking Questions and Seeking Clarifications

Strategies:

- Prepare a List of Questions: Before appointments, prepare a list of questions to ensure that all concerns are addressed during the limited time with healthcare professionals.
- Encourage Questions: Encourage healthcare providers to ask questions and seek clarifications to ensure mutual understanding.
- Utilize Educational Resources: Ask for educational resources or materials that can provide additional information about the cancer diagnosis, treatment options, and potential side effects.

Building a Trusting Relationship

Strategies:

- Establish Trust Early: Work on establishing trust early in the relationship with healthcare providers by being honest and transparent about symptoms, concerns, and preferences.
- Express Feelings and Concerns: Communicate openly about emotional concerns, fears, or anxieties related to the cancer journey, allowing healthcare professionals to provide appropriate support.
- Acknowledge Shared Decision-Making: Acknowledge and participate in shared decision-making processes, ensuring that personal values and preferences are considered in the treatment plan.

Advocating for Personalized Care

Strategies:

- Express Individual Preferences: Clearly communicate personal preferences regarding treatment options, involvement in decision-making, and the desired level of information.
- Discuss Quality of Life Priorities: Engage in discussions about quality of life priorities, including family responsibilities, work commitments, and personal goals.
- Ask About Alternative Treatments: Inquire about alternative or complementary treatments that align with personal preferences, seeking a comprehensive approach to care.

Clarifying Treatment Plans and Timelines

Strategies:

- Request a Clear Treatment Plan: Ensure that the healthcare team provides a clear and detailed treatment plan, including the goals, expected timeline, and potential side effects.
- Discuss Potential Complications: Address potential complications or challenges that may arise during treatment, allowing for proactive planning and management.
- Seek Regular Updates: Request regular updates on the progress of the treatment plan, any changes in medications, and adjustments to the overall care strategy.

Navigating Decision-Making Processes

Strategies:

- Participate Actively in Decisions: Actively participate in decisions about treatment options, procedures, and interventions, expressing personal preferences and concerns.
- Seek Second Opinions: If needed, seek second opinions from other healthcare professionals to gain different perspectives on the diagnosis and recommended treatments.
- Request Multidisciplinary Meetings: Advocate for multidisciplinary meetings where different specialists collaborate to optimize care and address complex cases.

Reporting Symptoms and Side Effects Promptly

Strategies:

- Maintain a Symptom Journal: Keep a journal of symptoms, side effects, and any changes in health to provide accurate and detailed information during healthcare appointments.
- Report Changes Promptly: Report any new or worsening symptoms promptly to the healthcare team, allowing for timely interventions and adjustments to the treatment plan.
- Utilize Telehealth Services: Take advantage of telehealth services for virtual consultations when physical presence is challenging, ensuring ongoing communication with healthcare providers.

Inquiring About Support Services and Resources

Strategies:

- Ask About Support Services: Inquire about available support services within the healthcare facility, such as counseling, nutritional support, or integrative therapies.
- Explore External Resources: Request information about external resources, including local support groups, cancer organizations, and community services that can complement the overall care plan.

- Clarify Insurance Coverage: Seek clarification on insurance coverage for support services, medications, and treatments to avoid unexpected financial burdens.

Addressing Emotional and Psychosocial Well-being

Strategies:

- Initiate Discussions About Well-being: Initiate conversations with healthcare providers about emotional well-being, stressors, and coping strategies.
- Request Referrals for Counseling: If needed, request referrals for counseling or psychosocial support services to address emotional challenges associated with the cancer journey.
- Discuss Impact on Family Dynamics: Engage in discussions about the impact of the cancer journey on family dynamics and relationships, exploring ways to provide comprehensive support.

Seeking Second Opinions When Necessary

Strategies:

- Express Intent to Seek Second Opinions: Communicate openly with the primary healthcare team about the intention to seek second opinions, emphasizing the collaborative nature of the decision.
- Ensure Efficient Information Transfer: Facilitate the efficient transfer of medical records, test results, and treatment plans to ensure that second opinion consultations are well-informed.
- Share Second Opinion Findings: Share the findings and recommendations from second opinions with the primary healthcare team, promoting a collaborative approach to care.

Chapter 6: Nutrition and Wellness during a Cancer Journey

Maintaining proper nutrition and overall wellness is crucial for moms undergoing a cancer journey. Adequate nutrition can support the body during treatment, aid in recovery, and contribute to overall well-being. This section provides strategies for moms to focus on nutrition and wellness during this challenging time.

Collaborating with a Registered Dietitian

Strategies:

- Request a Nutritional Assessment: Seek a nutritional assessment from a registered dietitian who specializes in cancer care to tailor dietary recommendations based on individual needs.
- Discuss Dietary Preferences: Communicate personal dietary preferences, restrictions, and cultural considerations to create a nutrition plan that aligns with individual choices.
- Explore Strategies for Maintaining Weight: If necessary, discuss strategies for maintaining weight during treatment, especially if there are concerns about weight loss.

Emphasizing a Balanced Diet

Strategies:

- Prioritize Fruits and Vegetables: Emphasize a variety of fruits and vegetables to ensure a rich intake of vitamins, minerals, and antioxidants.
- Incorporate Whole Grains: Choose whole grains such as brown rice, quinoa, and whole wheat to provide essential nutrients and dietary fiber.
- Include Lean Proteins: Include lean proteins, such as poultry, fish, beans, and tofu, to support muscle maintenance and immune function.
- Integrate Healthy Fats: Incorporate healthy fats from sources like avocados, nuts, seeds, and olive oil for essential fatty acids.

Managing Digestive Symptoms

Strategies:

- Modify Texture and Consistency: Adjust the texture and consistency of foods if experiencing difficulty swallowing or digestive issues. This may include incorporating soft or pureed foods.
- Stay Hydrated: Maintain proper hydration by consuming water, herbal teas, or diluted fruit juices throughout the day to support digestion and prevent dehydration.
- Opt for Small, Frequent Meals: Choose small, frequent meals rather than large meals to manage digestive symptoms and maintain energy levels.

Addressing Changes in Taste and Smell

Strategies:

- Experiment with Flavors: Experiment with various herbs, spices, and seasonings to enhance the flavor of foods, especially if there are changes in taste perception.
- Opt for Cold or Room Temperature Foods: Cold or room temperature foods may be more palatable for those experiencing alterations in taste and smell.
- Balance Temperature and Texture: Balance the temperature and texture of foods to find combinations that are more appealing during treatment.

Ensuring Adequate Caloric Intake

Strategies:

- Choose Nutrient-Dense Foods: Focus on nutrient-dense foods to ensure the intake of essential vitamins and minerals despite potential challenges in appetite.
- Include High-Calorie Snacks: Incorporate high-calorie snacks, such as nuts, dried fruits, and energy-dense smoothies, to boost overall caloric intake.
- Consult with a Dietitian: Work with a registered dietitian to calculate and monitor caloric needs, especially if there are concerns about unintentional weight loss.

Supplements and Nutritional Support

Strategies:

- Consult Healthcare Team: Consult with healthcare professionals, including oncologists and dietitians, before incorporating nutritional supplements to address specific deficiencies.
- Consider Multivitamins: If recommended by healthcare providers, consider taking a multivitamin to supplement any nutrient gaps in the diet.
- Discuss Nutritional Drinks: Explore nutritional drinks or shakes recommended by healthcare professionals to supplement caloric and nutrient intake.

Managing Side Effects of Treatment

Strategies:

- Address Nausea: Choose easily digestible foods and separate liquids from solids to help manage nausea. Ginger and peppermint may also offer relief.
- Stay Hydrated During Diarrhea: Consume electrolyte-rich beverages and incorporate binding foods (such as bananas and rice) to manage diarrhea and prevent dehydration.

- Adjust Diet for Mouth Sores: Opt for soft, bland foods and avoid acidic or spicy items if experiencing mouth sores. Maintaining good oral hygiene is crucial during this time.

Prioritizing Hydration

Strategies:

- Regularly Consume Fluids: Aim to consume an adequate amount of fluids throughout the day, including water, herbal teas, and clear broths.
- Monitor Hydration Status: Monitor hydration status by paying attention to urine color and frequency, ensuring it remains light yellow or pale.
- Seek Fluid-Rich Foods: Incorporate fluid-rich foods like fruits (watermelon, oranges) and vegetables (cucumbers, celery) into the diet.

Encouraging Physical Activity

Strategies:

- Consult with Healthcare Team: Obtain clearance from healthcare professionals before starting or modifying an exercise routine, taking into account individual health status and treatment plan.
- Choose Gentle Activities: Opt for gentle exercises such as walking, yoga, or swimming, adjusting intensity based on energy levels and overall well-being.
- Prioritize Flexibility and Strength: Include activities that focus on flexibility and strength to support overall physical health and mitigate treatment-related fatigue.

Prioritizing Emotional and Mental Well-being

Strategies:

- Incorporate Relaxation Techniques: Practice relaxation techniques such as deep breathing, meditation, or mindfulness to manage stress and promote mental well-being.
- Engage in Activities for Joy: Participate in activities that bring joy and relaxation, whether it's reading, listening to music, or spending time in nature.
- Seek Professional Support: If needed, seek support from mental health professionals or counselors to address emotional challenges and coping strategies.

Individualizing Nutrition Plans

Importance:

- Tailoring to Personal Preferences: Individualized nutrition plans take into account personal dietary preferences, cultural considerations, and specific needs, ensuring a more personalized and sustainable approach.
- Catering to Treatment Modalities: Different cancer treatments may have varied effects on appetite, taste, and digestion. Individualized nutrition plans can be adjusted to accommodate these specific challenges.

Collaborating with Healthcare Professionals

Importance:

- Informed Decision-Making: Working with healthcare professionals, including registered dietitians, ensures that nutrition plans are informed by medical history, treatment protocols, and individual needs.
- Addressing Specialized Needs: Some cancer treatments may necessitate specialized nutrition interventions. Collaborating with healthcare professionals helps address these specific needs.

Promoting Long-Term Health and Survivorship

Importance:

- Establishing Healthy Habits: Embracing a balanced and nutritious diet during treatment sets the foundation for long-term health and survivorship.
- Reducing Long-Term Risks: Proper nutrition may contribute to reducing the risk of long-term complications or secondary health issues that can arise post-treatment.

Exercise and Physical Well-being During a Cancer Journey

Incorporating exercise into the routine during a cancer journey can have numerous physical and emotional benefits. While individual abilities and preferences vary, engaging in appropriate physical activity can enhance overall well-being, improve energy levels, and contribute to a sense of empowerment. This section provides strategies for moms to prioritize exercise and maintain physical well-being during their cancer journey.

Consultation with Healthcare Professionals

Strategies:

- Seek Medical Clearance: Obtain medical clearance from healthcare professionals, ensuring that exercise is safe and suitable based on individual health conditions and treatment plans.
- Collaborate with Rehabilitation Specialists: If applicable, collaborate with rehabilitation specialists, such as physical therapists or occupational therapists, to design a tailored exercise plan that considers any physical limitations.

Choosing Suitable Types of Exercise

Strategies:

- Low-Impact Activities: Opt for low-impact activities such as walking, swimming, or stationary cycling, which are gentle on the joints and muscles.
- Adapt to Energy Levels: Modify the intensity and duration of exercise based on energy levels and overall well-being, allowing for flexibility in the routine.
- Incorporate Enjoyable Activities: Choose exercises that are enjoyable, making it more likely to stick to the routine. This could include activities like dancing, yoga, or gardening.

Setting Realistic Goals

Strategies:

- Establish Realistic Goals: Set achievable and realistic exercise goals, considering individual fitness levels, treatment-related side effects, and daily responsibilities.
- Focus on Consistency: Emphasize consistency over intensity, aiming for regular, moderate exercise rather than sporadic intense sessions.
- Celebrate Small Achievements: Celebrate small achievements and milestones, recognizing the positive impact of regular physical activity on overall well-being.

Prioritizing Flexibility and Strength Training

Strategies:

- Incorporate Stretching Exercises: Include flexibility exercises, such as stretching routines or yoga, to maintain joint mobility and reduce muscle tension.
- Include Strength Training: Incorporate light resistance training to maintain or improve muscle strength, focusing on major muscle groups. This can be done using resistance bands, bodyweight exercises, or light weights.

Listening to the Body

Strategies:

- Practice Mindful Movement: Engage in mindful movement, paying attention to how the body feels during and after exercise, and adjusting activities accordingly.
- Rest and Recovery: Allow for adequate rest and recovery between exercise sessions, especially on days when fatigue or other treatment-related side effects are more pronounced.
- Modify as Needed: Be open to modifying the exercise routine based on changing circumstances, such as treatment schedules, energy levels, or physical symptoms.

Engaging in Supportive Activities

Strategies:

- Join Exercise Classes: Participate in cancer-specific exercise classes or support group activities that cater to individuals undergoing similar journeys, providing a sense of community.
- Involve Family and Friends: Include family members or friends in physical activities to enhance motivation and create a supportive environment.
- Explore Mind-Body Practices: Explore mind-body practices such as tai chi or meditation, which not only contribute to physical well-being but also address emotional and mental health.

Maintaining Hydration and Nutrition

Strategies:

- Stay Hydrated: Prioritize hydration before, during, and after exercise, especially important during cancer treatment when hydration needs may be increased.
- Support with Nutrient-Rich Foods: Consume nutrient-rich foods to support energy levels and aid in recovery after exercise. A well-balanced diet contributes to overall physical well-being.

Adapting to Treatment Phases

Strategies:

- Adjust During Active Treatment: Modify exercise routines during active treatment phases to accommodate fluctuations in energy levels, potential side effects, and medical recommendations.

- Gradual Reintroduction Post-Treatment: After completing treatment, gradually reintroduce or adjust exercise routines, taking into account recovery and any lasting effects of treatment.

Seeking Professional Guidance

Strategies:

- Consult with Exercise Specialists: Consult with exercise specialists, such as certified trainers or physical therapists with experience in cancer care, for personalized guidance.
- Explore Rehabilitation Programs: Explore rehabilitation programs designed for cancer survivors, offering structured and supervised exercise sessions in a supportive environment.
- Incorporate Therapeutic Modalities: Consider incorporating therapeutic modalities such as hydrotherapy or gentle massage, under professional guidance, to complement physical well-being.

Monitoring Mental Well-being

Strategies:

- Recognize Emotional Benefits: Acknowledge and appreciate the emotional benefits of exercise, such as reduced stress, improved mood, and enhanced overall mental well-being.
- Address Anxiety and Depression: If dealing with anxiety or depression, consider exercises known for their positive impact on mental health, such as aerobic activities, yoga, or mindfulness practices.
- Seek Professional Support: If needed, seek support from mental health professionals to address emotional challenges and integrate holistic strategies for well-being.

Integrative Therapies for Well-being During a Cancer Journey

Integrative therapies encompass a range of complementary approaches that can enhance the overall well-being of individuals undergoing a cancer journey. These therapies, when used alongside conventional medical treatments, may help manage symptoms, improve quality of life, and provide emotional and physical support. This section explores various integrative therapies that moms can consider during their cancer journey.

Mind-Body Practices

Therapies:

- Mindfulness Meditation: Engage in mindfulness meditation to cultivate awareness, reduce stress, and enhance emotional well-being.

- Guided Imagery: Practice guided imagery exercises to promote relaxation, manage anxiety, and foster a positive mindset.
- Deep Breathing Techniques: Incorporate deep breathing exercises to alleviate stress, improve oxygenation, and enhance overall respiratory function.

Acupuncture and Acupressure

Therapies:

- Acupuncture: Consider acupuncture, a traditional Chinese medicine practice involving the insertion of thin needles into specific points on the body, to help manage symptoms such as pain, nausea, and fatigue.
- Acupressure: Explore acupressure, a technique that involves applying pressure to specific points on the body, as a non-invasive alternative to acupuncture.

Massage Therapy

Therapies:

- Swedish Massage: Opt for Swedish massage to promote relaxation, improve circulation, and alleviate muscle tension.
- Manual Lymphatic Drainage: Consider manual lymphatic drainage for individuals experiencing lymphedema, a gentle massage technique aimed at reducing swelling.

Yoga and Tai Chi

Therapies:

- Yoga: Practice yoga for its physical and mental benefits, including improved flexibility, strength, and stress reduction. Adaptive yoga classes are available to accommodate various fitness levels.
- Tai Chi: Engage in tai chi, a Chinese martial art characterized by slow, flowing movements, to enhance balance, flexibility, and overall well-being.

Herbal Supplements and Nutritional Support

Therapies:

- Consult with Healthcare Professionals: Prior to incorporating herbal supplements, consult with healthcare professionals to ensure they do not interfere with conventional treatments and are safe for individual health conditions.

- Nutritional Support: Explore nutritional supplements, under the guidance of healthcare providers or registered dietitians, to address specific nutrient needs and support overall health.

Aromatherapy

Therapies:

- Essential Oils: Use essential oils through aromatherapy to promote relaxation, alleviate nausea, and improve mood. Certain scents, such as lavender and peppermint, are commonly used for their calming effects.

Art and Music Therapy

Therapies:

- Art Therapy: Engage in art therapy as a creative outlet for expression and emotional processing. This can involve drawing, painting, or other artistic activities.
- Music Therapy: Explore music therapy to enhance emotional well-being, reduce stress, and promote relaxation. Listening to preferred music or learning to play an instrument can be therapeutic.

Supportive Counseling and Psychotherapy

Therapies:

- Individual Counseling: Seek individual counseling or psychotherapy to address emotional challenges, cope with stress, and navigate the complexities of the cancer journey.
- Group Therapy: Participate in group therapy sessions to connect with others facing similar experiences, share insights, and gain mutual support.

Exercise and Physical Activity

Therapies:

- Adaptive Exercise Programs: Engage in adaptive exercise programs designed for individuals undergoing cancer treatment. These programs may include modified workouts tailored to individual fitness levels.

- Outdoor Activities: Explore outdoor activities such as nature walks, gardening, or gentle hikes to combine physical activity with the therapeutic benefits of spending time in nature.

Journaling and Expressive Writing

Therapies:

- Journaling: Keep a journal to express thoughts, emotions, and reflections throughout the cancer journey. Writing can be a cathartic and reflective practice.
- Expressive Writing: Consider participating in guided expressive writing exercises, focusing on the emotional aspects of the cancer experience.

Educational and Supportive Programs

Therapies:

- Attend Workshops and Seminars: Attend educational workshops or seminars focused on integrative therapies, providing insights into various approaches and empowering individuals with knowledge.
- Join Supportive Programs: Explore structured programs that combine multiple integrative therapies, offering a holistic approach to well-being.

Incorporating Mindful Eating Practices

Therapies:

- Mindful Eating: Practice mindful eating to enhance the connection between food and well-being. Pay attention to flavors, textures, and the overall experience of eating, promoting a positive relationship with food.

Balancing Rest and Activity

Strategies:

- Prioritize Rest: Recognize the importance of rest and allow for adequate periods of relaxation between activities and therapies.
- Listen to the Body: Pay attention to the body's signals and adjust the intensity and frequency of integrative therapies based on individual energy levels and overall well-being.

Collaborating with Healthcare Professionals

Strategies:

- Inform Healthcare Team: Communicate openly with healthcare professionals about the integration of complementary therapies into the overall care plan, ensuring alignment with medical treatments.
- Seek Guidance: Consult with healthcare providers or integrative medicine specialists for guidance on the most suitable therapies based on individual health conditions and treatment protocols.

Chapter 7: Caring for the Caregivers: Supporting Moms in Their Cancer Journey

Caregivers play a crucial role in providing emotional, physical, and practical support to moms undergoing a cancer journey. It is essential to recognize the challenges faced by caregivers and offer strategies to enhance their well-being. This section focuses on caring for the caregivers, providing guidance and support to those who are dedicating themselves to supporting moms through the challenges of cancer.

Acknowledging Caregiver's Role and Feelings

Strategies:

- Express Gratitude: Acknowledge and express gratitude for the caregiver's dedication, recognizing the vital role they play in supporting the mom through the cancer journey.
- Encourage Open Communication: Create an environment where caregivers feel comfortable expressing their feelings, concerns, and needs.

Building a Support Network for Caregivers

Strategies:

- Encourage Connections: Facilitate connections between caregivers facing similar challenges. Support groups or online forums provide spaces for sharing experiences and offering mutual support.
- Involve Family and Friends: Encourage the involvement of family and friends in providing additional assistance and emotional support.

Providing Respite Care

Strategies:

- Arrange Breaks: Organize scheduled breaks for caregivers to rest and recharge. This can involve enlisting the help of other family members, friends, or professional respite care services.
- Offer Flexibility: Provide flexibility in caregiving responsibilities, allowing caregivers to balance their own needs with the demands of caregiving.

Addressing Caregiver's Physical Well-being

Strategies:

- Encourage Self-Care Practices: Advocate for self-care practices, including regular exercise, proper nutrition, and sufficient sleep, to support the caregiver's physical well-being.
- Promote Healthcare Check-ups: Encourage caregivers to attend regular healthcare check-ups to monitor their own health and address any emerging concerns.

Managing Caregiver Stress and Anxiety

Strategies:

- Provide Stress-Reduction Techniques: Offer stress-reduction techniques such as mindfulness, deep breathing exercises, or guided relaxation to help caregivers manage anxiety.
- Suggest Professional Support: Recommend professional counseling or support groups where caregivers can explore their emotions and receive guidance on managing stress.

Offering Practical Assistance

Strategies:

- Coordinate Practical Support: Organize practical assistance, such as meal deliveries, transportation help, or assistance with household chores, to lighten the caregiver's load.
- Identify Community Resources: Connect caregivers with local community resources and services that can provide additional practical support.

Fostering Emotional Support for Caregivers

Strategies:

- Encourage Emotional Expression: Create an atmosphere where caregivers feel comfortable expressing their emotions. This can involve journaling, talking with friends, or seeking professional counseling.
- Validate Feelings: Acknowledge the validity of the caregiver's feelings and provide reassurance that experiencing a range of emotions is a normal part of the caregiving journey.

Supporting Work-Life Balance

Strategies:

- Flexible Work Arrangements: Advocate for flexible work arrangements for caregivers who are also managing employment responsibilities. This may include modified schedules or remote work options.
- Explore Employer Resources: Identify and explore resources provided by employers, such as employee assistance programs (EAPs) or workplace support services.

Facilitating Open Communication

Strategies:

- Regular Check-Ins: Schedule regular check-ins with caregivers to discuss their well-being, assess needs, and address any emerging challenges.
- Provide Information: Keep caregivers informed about the mom's health status, treatment plans, and any changes in caregiving responsibilities.

Respecting Caregiver's Autonomy

Strategies:

- Respect Decision-Making: Acknowledge and respect the caregiver's role in decision-making processes, allowing them to actively participate in discussions about the mom's care.
- Provide Information and Options: Ensure that caregivers have access to relevant information and options related to the mom's treatment and care, allowing them to make informed decisions.

Celebrating Caregiver Milestones

Strategies:

- Acknowledge Achievements: Celebrate caregiver milestones and accomplishments, whether they relate to caregiving tasks, personal goals, or self-care achievements.
- Express Appreciation: Regularly express appreciation for the caregiver's dedication, effort, and resilience throughout the cancer journey.

Encouraging Caregiver-Boundaries

Strategies:

- Set Clear Boundaries: Encourage caregivers to set clear boundaries on their time, energy, and emotional resources. Establishing boundaries helps prevent burnout and promotes sustainable caregiving.
- Provide Alternatives: Offer alternative solutions when caregivers need to step back temporarily, ensuring that other support systems are in place.

Planning for Transitions in Care

Strategies:

- Facilitate Care Transition Planning: Plan for transitions in care, especially if the mom's treatment plan evolves or if there are changes in caregiving responsibilities. Ensure clear communication and support during these transitions.
- Coordinate with Healthcare Team: Collaborate with the healthcare team to ensure a smooth transition and provide caregivers with the necessary information and resources.

Recognizing and Addressing Caregiver Grief

Strategies:

- Acknowledge Grief: Recognize that caregivers may experience grief and loss throughout the cancer journey. Encourage open conversations about these feelings and provide avenues for support.
- Connect with Bereavement Services: If the cancer journey takes a difficult turn, connect caregivers with bereavement services and support groups to help them navigate the grieving process.

Encouraging Caregiver Self-Reflection

Strategies:

- Promote Self-Reflection: Encourage caregivers to engage in self-reflection to understand their evolving needs, emotions, and coping strategies. Self-awareness can contribute to more effective caregiving.
- Explore Personal Growth Opportunities: Support caregivers in exploring personal growth opportunities, whether through educational pursuits, hobbies, or activities that bring personal fulfillment.

Recognizing and Addressing Caregiver Burnout

Caregiver burnout is a common challenge faced by individuals providing care to loved ones, particularly during a demanding and emotionally charged situation like a cancer journey. It is crucial to recognize the signs of burnout and implement strategies to prevent and address it effectively. This section outlines key considerations for recognizing and addressing caregiver burnout, with a focus on supporting those caring for moms undergoing a cancer journey.

Signs of Caregiver Burnout

Signs to Watch for:

- Physical Exhaustion: Constant fatigue, sleep disturbances, and persistent physical ailments.
- Emotional Exhaustion: Feelings of overwhelming sadness, irritability, or a sense of hopelessness.
- Withdrawal: Social isolation, withdrawal from activities once enjoyed, or strained relationships with family and friends.
- Decreased Immune Function: Frequent illnesses or a decline in overall immune system function.
- Impaired Concentration: Difficulty focusing, forgetfulness, or diminished cognitive function.
- Neglecting Personal Needs: Ignoring one's own physical and emotional needs, including healthcare appointments and self-care practices.
- Loss of Interest: A diminished interest in hobbies, activities, or personal goals.
- Increased Irritability: Heightened irritability, impatience, or an inability to cope with stressors.
- Changes in Sleep or Eating Patterns: Disruptions in sleep patterns, changes in appetite, or weight fluctuations.
- Feeling Overwhelmed: A constant sense of being overwhelmed by caregiving responsibilities.

Strategies for Addressing Caregiver Burnout

Intervention Strategies:

- Encourage Self-Reflection: Prompt caregivers to reflect on their own well-being, acknowledging the challenges they face and recognizing signs of burnout.
- Open Communication: Create a safe space for caregivers to openly discuss their feelings, concerns, and experiences. Ensure they feel heard and understood.
- Normalize Help-Seeking: Reinforce that seeking help is not a sign of weakness but a necessary step in maintaining one's well-being.
- Education on Burnout: Provide information and resources that help caregivers understand the concept of burnout, its signs, and the importance of proactive intervention.
- Professional Support: Encourage caregivers to seek professional support through counseling, therapy, or support groups to address emotional challenges and learn coping strategies.
- Respite Care: Facilitate respite care to give caregivers breaks from their responsibilities, allowing them to rest and recharge.
- Empower with Information: Provide caregivers with information about available support services, community resources, and caregiver assistance programs.
- Share Responsibilities: Help distribute caregiving responsibilities among family members and friends to prevent one individual from bearing the entire burden.
- Set Realistic Expectations: Work with caregivers to establish realistic expectations for their role, helping them understand their limits and prioritize self-care.
- Encourage Boundaries: Support caregivers in setting clear boundaries on their time and energy, emphasizing the importance of self-preservation.
- Celebrate Small Wins: Acknowledge and celebrate small achievements and milestones, reinforcing the value of the caregiver's efforts.
- Promote Physical Well-being: Advocate for caregivers to prioritize their physical health through regular exercise, proper nutrition, and adequate sleep.
- Connect with Peers: Facilitate connections between caregivers who can share experiences, insights, and coping strategies. Peer support can be invaluable.
- Engage in Relaxation Techniques: Introduce relaxation techniques such as deep breathing, meditation, or mindfulness to help caregivers manage stress and promote emotional well-being.
- Address Guilt: Recognize and address any feelings of guilt caregivers may experience, emphasizing that self-care is not a selfish act but a necessary one.
- Involve Healthcare Professionals: Encourage caregivers to communicate openly with the healthcare team, seeking guidance and support for both the mom and themselves.
- Plan for Resilience: Help caregivers develop resilience strategies, emphasizing the importance of adapting to challenges and bouncing back from difficult situations.

Preventive Strategies:

- Early Intervention: Recognize signs of stress and burnout early on, intervening proactively to prevent escalating challenges.
- Regular Check-Ins: Establish a routine of regular check-ins to assess the caregiver's well-being and provide support before burnout becomes severe.
- Education on Self-Care: Educate caregivers on the importance of consistent self-care practices and assist them in developing self-care routines.
- Stress Reduction Techniques: Promote stress reduction techniques, including exercise, meditation, and hobbies, to help caregivers manage stress proactively.
- Resilience Building: Provide resources and activities that promote resilience, helping caregivers build coping mechanisms for navigating the ups and downs of caregiving.
- Community Engagement: Encourage involvement in community groups or activities that provide social support and opportunities for shared experiences.

Self-Care Strategies for Moms During a Cancer Journey

Self-care is essential for moms undergoing a cancer journey, as it helps nurture their physical, emotional, and mental well-being. Taking intentional steps to prioritize self-care can contribute to resilience, improved coping, and an enhanced sense of well-being. This section outlines various self-care strategies specifically tailored to support moms facing the challenges of cancer.

Prioritizing Emotional Well-being

Strategies:

- Expressive Writing: Engage in expressive writing as a way to process emotions, thoughts, and reflections about the cancer journey.
- Mindfulness Practices: Practice mindfulness through meditation, deep breathing exercises, or guided imagery to promote emotional balance and reduce stress.
- Therapeutic Activities: Participate in therapeutic activities such as art or music therapy to express emotions and find comfort in creative expression.
- Emotional Support: Seek and maintain emotional support through friends, family, or support groups, fostering connections with those who understand the unique challenges of a cancer journey.

Nurturing Physical Well-being

Strategies:

- Gentle Exercise: Engage in gentle exercises such as walking, yoga, or swimming to maintain physical well-being and alleviate stress.
- Adequate Rest: Prioritize adequate rest and sleep, recognizing the importance of allowing the body time to recover.
- Balanced Nutrition: Maintain a balanced and nutritious diet, incorporating a variety of foods that support overall health and energy levels.
- Hydration: Stay well-hydrated to support bodily functions and counteract potential effects of cancer treatments.

Managing Practical Matters

Strategies:

- Delegating Tasks: Delegate household tasks and responsibilities to family members or friends to alleviate the burden on personal time and energy.
- Organizational Tools: Use organizational tools such as calendars or apps to help manage appointments, treatment schedules, and other logistical aspects of the cancer journey.
- Time Management: Prioritize tasks and manage time effectively, recognizing when to ask for assistance and when to take breaks.

Cultivating Relaxation and Stress Reduction

Strategies:

- Relaxation Techniques: Incorporate relaxation techniques such as warm baths, aromatherapy, or guided relaxation to reduce stress and promote a sense of calm.
- Nature Connection: Spend time in nature, whether through short walks, gardening, or simply enjoying outdoor spaces, to enhance well-being and reduce stress.
- Hobbies and Interests: Engage in hobbies and activities that bring joy and relaxation, providing an outlet for self-expression and creativity.

Addressing Social and Relationship Needs

Strategies:

- Maintaining Connections: Prioritize maintaining connections with friends and loved ones, both in-person and virtually, to foster a supportive network.

- Date Nights or Outings: Plan occasional date nights or outings with a partner or close friends to create moments of joy and relaxation.
- Open Communication: Communicate openly with family and friends about personal needs and boundaries, allowing for a supportive and understanding network.

Seeking Professional Support

Strategies:

- Counseling or Therapy: Consider individual or family counseling to address emotional challenges, provide coping strategies, and strengthen resilience.
- Supportive Services: Explore support services offered by cancer centers, including social workers, psychologists, or counselors who specialize in cancer-related issues.

Personal Reflection and Mindful Moments

Strategies:

- Daily Reflection: Incorporate daily moments of reflection, whether through journaling, meditation, or quiet contemplation, to check in with personal emotions and needs.
- Mindful Moments: Integrate mindful moments into daily routines, savoring small joys, and being present in the moment.

Balancing Personal and Family Needs

Strategies:

- Communicate Boundaries: Clearly communicate personal boundaries and needs to family members, ensuring an understanding of the importance of self-care.
- Scheduling "Me Time": Schedule dedicated "me time" in the daily or weekly routine to focus on personal interests or relaxation.

Creative Outlets and Self-Expression

Strategies:

- Creative Expression: Explore creative outlets such as writing, art, or music to express emotions and tap into personal sources of strength and resilience.
- Self-Expression: Embrace opportunities for self-expression, whether through fashion, personal style, or other outlets that reflect individual identity.

Celebrating Milestones and Achievements

Strategies:

- Acknowledge Achievements: Celebrate personal milestones, no matter how small, to recognize and appreciate personal resilience and growth.
- Positive Reinforcement: Offer positive reinforcement and self-encouragement, cultivating a mindset that focuses on progress and personal strength.

Spiritual and Mind-Body Connection

Strategies:

- Spiritual Practices: Engage in spiritual practices that bring comfort and connection, such as prayer, meditation, or participation in religious or spiritual communities.
- Mind-Body Techniques: Explore mind-body techniques like tai chi or qi gong to enhance the connection between mental and physical well-being.

Continuing Education and Personal Growth

Strategies:

- Online Courses or Workshops: Explore online courses or workshops in areas of personal interest or growth to nurture intellectual well-being.
- Book Clubs or Learning Groups: Join book clubs or learning groups to engage with new ideas and perspectives, fostering continuous personal development.

Building a Support Network

Strategies:

- Joining Support Groups: Consider joining cancer-specific support groups or communities to connect with others facing similar challenges and share experiences.
- Networking with Other Moms: Connect with other moms going through a cancer journey, either locally or online, to build a supportive network of understanding peers.

Professional Development and Career Planning

Strategies:

- Professional Development: Explore opportunities for professional development or career planning, considering long-term goals and aspirations.
- Flexible Work Arrangements: If applicable, discuss flexible work arrangements with employers to create a supportive and manageable work-life balance.

*32.15 Planning for Future and Legacy**

Strategies:

- Legacy Projects: Consider engaging in projects that contribute to a personal legacy, such as creating family traditions, documenting personal stories, or leaving messages for loved ones.
- Future Planning: When ready, engage in future planning discussions, addressing personal wishes, and ensuring a sense of control over future aspects of life.

Chapter 8: Survivorship and Life After Cancer: A New Beginning

Survivorship marks the transition from active cancer treatment to the phase of life beyond cancer. This period involves a shift in focus from medical interventions to rebuilding and embracing a new sense of normalcy. This section explores various aspects of survivorship and offers guidance for individuals, including moms, as they navigate life after cancer.

Embracing the Survivor Identity

Strategies:

- Self-Reflection: Take time for self-reflection to embrace and internalize the identity of a cancer survivor, acknowledging the strength and resilience demonstrated throughout the journey.
- Celebrate Milestones: Celebrate survivorship milestones, recognizing the achievements and progress made since the initial diagnosis and treatment.

Managing Fear of Recurrence

Strategies:

- Open Dialogue with Healthcare Team: Engage in open dialogues with healthcare providers about fears of recurrence, discussing any symptoms or concerns promptly.
- Counseling Support: Seek counseling support to address anxiety or fear of recurrence, developing coping strategies to manage these emotions.

Navigating Changes in Body Image

Strategies:

- Body Image Acceptance: Embrace changes in body image, acknowledging the strength and resilience reflected in the body's journey through cancer.
- Clothing and Appearance Choices: Make choices regarding clothing and appearance that align with personal comfort and self-expression.

Reintegration into Daily Life

Strategies:

- Goal Setting: Set realistic goals for personal and professional endeavors, recognizing the importance of gradual reintegration into daily life.
- Adapting to Changes: Adapt to any changes in priorities, perspectives, or life goals that may have emerged during the cancer journey.

Future Planning and Goal Setting

Strategies:

- Setting Future Goals: Engage in future planning and goal setting, focusing on personal aspirations, relationships, and endeavors that bring joy and fulfillment.
- Pursuing Personal Interests: Explore personal interests and hobbies, using this time to pursue activities that contribute to overall life satisfaction.

Advocacy and Giving Back

Strategies:

- Advocacy Opportunities: Consider advocacy opportunities or involvement in cancer-related causes, contributing to awareness, support, and positive change.
- Sharing Experiences: Share personal experiences with others, offering support and insights to individuals currently navigating the challenges of a cancer diagnosis.

Maintaining Health Surveillance and Preventive Care

Strategies:

- Adhering to Preventive Measures: Adhere to recommended preventive measures, including vaccinations, screenings, and lifestyle choices that contribute to long-term health.
- Health Surveillance: Remain vigilant about health surveillance, promptly addressing any concerns or symptoms that may arise.

Transitioning to Life After Cancer Treatment: Navigating the Next Chapter

Transitioning from active cancer treatment to life after treatment is a significant milestone that comes with its own set of challenges and adjustments. This phase involves rebuilding and adapting to a new normalcy. Here are essential considerations and strategies for individuals, including moms, as they navigate the transition to life after cancer treatment.

*34.1 Post-Treatment Follow-Up and Monitoring**

Strategies:

- Regular Follow-Up Appointments: Attend scheduled follow-up appointments with healthcare professionals to monitor overall health, address lingering concerns, and ensure a smooth transition to post-treatment life.
- Health Surveillance: Be vigilant about personal health, promptly reporting any new symptoms or changes to the healthcare team.

*34.2 Emotional Well-being and Mental Health**

Strategies:

- Continued Emotional Support: Maintain connections with support systems, whether through friends, family, or support groups, to navigate emotional challenges that may arise post-treatment.
- Counseling or Therapy: Consider ongoing counseling or therapy to address emotional aspects of the cancer journey and support mental well-being.
- Mindfulness Practices: Integrate mindfulness practices into daily life to promote emotional balance and cope with stressors.

*34.3 Physical Wellness and Lifestyle Choices**

Strategies:

- Gradual Physical Activity: Gradually reintroduce physical activity into daily life, starting with gentle exercises and progressing based on individual capabilities.
- Nutritious Diet: Maintain a nutritious and balanced diet, focusing on foods that support overall health and recovery.
- Hydration: Stay well-hydrated to support bodily functions and aid in the recovery process.
- Sleep Hygiene: Prioritize healthy sleep habits to support physical and mental well-being.

*34.4 Managing Post-Treatment Symptoms**

Strategies:

- Open Communication with Healthcare Team: Communicate openly with healthcare providers about any post-treatment symptoms or side effects, seeking guidance on managing and addressing these concerns.
- Symptom Management Techniques: Explore symptom management techniques, whether through medications, lifestyle adjustments, or complementary therapies.

*34.5 Relationship Dynamics and Support Systems**

Strategies:

- Reconnecting with Loved Ones: Reconnect with loved ones and rebuild relationships that may have been impacted during the treatment phase, emphasizing open communication and shared experiences.
- Support System Strengthening: Strengthen support systems by engaging with friends, family, and support groups that understand and appreciate the post-treatment journey.

*34.6 Reproductive and Sexual Health Considerations**

Strategies:

- Reproductive Health Discussions: Engage in discussions about reproductive health, including family planning, fertility considerations, and any potential impacts of cancer treatment on these aspects.
- Consulting Specialists: Consult reproductive specialists if there are specific concerns or questions regarding fertility or sexual health post-treatment.

*34.7 Employment and Vocational Considerations**

Strategies:

- Return to Work Planning: If applicable, plan the return to work gradually, taking into account individual energy levels and adjusting responsibilities as needed.
- Communication with Employers: Communicate openly with employers about any necessary workplace accommodations or modifications.

*34.8 Financial and Legal Aspects**

Strategies:

- Financial Review: Review financial considerations post-treatment, including insurance coverage, potential changes in employment, and any adjustments needed for financial stability.
- Legal Documentation Updates: Update legal documents, such as wills, advance directives, and power of attorney, to reflect current wishes and preferences.

*34.9 Reintegration into Daily Life and Routine**

Strategies:

- Gradual Reintegration: Gradually reintegrate into daily life and routines, recognizing that adjustments may be necessary based on energy levels and personal capabilities.
- Time Management: Implement effective time management strategies to balance personal needs, work responsibilities, and leisure activities.

*34.10 Survivorship Care Plans and Healthcare Navigation**

Strategies:

- Survivorship Care Plan Utilization: Leverage the survivorship care plan developed in collaboration with healthcare providers to guide post-treatment care and address ongoing healthcare needs.
- Healthcare Navigation: Navigate the healthcare system effectively, understanding the availability of resources, support services, and survivorship programs.

*34.11 Addressing Fear of Recurrence and Anxiety**

Strategies:

- Open Dialogue with Healthcare Team: Engage in open dialogues with healthcare providers about fears of recurrence, discussing any symptoms or concerns promptly.
- Counseling Support: Seek counseling support to address anxiety or fear of recurrence, developing coping strategies to manage these emotions.

*34.12 Reconnecting with Hobbies and Interests**

Strategies:

- Hobbies and Activities: Reconnect with hobbies and activities that bring joy and fulfillment, fostering a sense of personal enjoyment and accomplishment.
- Exploration of New Interests: Explore new interests or activities that align with post-treatment goals and aspirations.

*34.13 Future Planning and Goal Setting**

Strategies:

- Setting Post-Treatment Goals: Engage in future planning and goal setting, focusing on personal aspirations, relationships, and endeavors that contribute to overall life satisfaction.
- Pursuing Personal and Professional Growth: Explore opportunities for personal and professional growth, embracing new challenges and experiences.

*34.14 Advocacy and Sharing Experiences**

Strategies:

- Advocacy Involvement: Consider involvement in advocacy opportunities or activities related to cancer awareness and support.
- Sharing Experiences: Share personal experiences with others, providing insights and support to individuals currently navigating the challenges of life after cancer treatment.

*34.15 Maintaining Health Surveillance and Preventive Care**

Strategies:

- Adhering to Preventive Measures: Adhere to recommended preventive measures, including vaccinations, screenings, and lifestyle choices that contribute to long-term health.
- Health Surveillance: Remain vigilant about health surveillance, promptly addressing any concerns or symptoms that may arise.

Follow-up Care and Monitoring: Nurturing Well-being Beyond Treatment Completion

As individuals transition to life after cancer treatment, follow-up care and monitoring play a crucial role in maintaining overall well-being and detecting any potential issues early. This phase involves ongoing medical check-ups, surveillance, and self-care practices. Here's a comprehensive guide to follow-up care and monitoring:

1. **Regular Medical Check-ups:**

- Schedule regular follow-up appointments with your oncologist or healthcare team as recommended. These appointments are essential for monitoring your health and addressing any concerns that may arise.

2. Surveillance and Imaging:

- Depending on the type of cancer and treatment received, your healthcare team may recommend periodic imaging tests, such as CT scans, MRIs, or PET scans, to monitor for any signs of recurrence or new developments.

3. Blood Tests:

- Routine blood tests may be conducted to assess various markers and indicators, providing insights into your overall health and detecting any abnormalities.

4. Physical Examinations:

- Physical examinations by healthcare professionals are vital for identifying any physical changes or symptoms that may require further investigation.

5. Survivorship Care Plans:

- Work with your healthcare team to develop a survivorship care plan. This personalized document outlines your treatment history, potential long-term effects, and recommendations for ongoing care and monitoring.

6. Emotional and Mental Well-being:

- Prioritize your emotional and mental well-being. Consider engaging in counseling, support groups, or other mental health services to address any lingering emotional challenges.

7. **Healthy Lifestyle Practices:**

- Maintain a healthy lifestyle by incorporating regular exercise, a balanced diet, and sufficient sleep. These practices contribute to overall well-being and may reduce the risk of certain health issues.

8. **Early Detection of Potential Issues:**

- Be vigilant about changes in your body and promptly report any new symptoms or concerns to your healthcare team. Early detection is key to addressing potential issues promptly.

9. **Communication with Healthcare Professionals:**

- Foster open and transparent communication with your healthcare team. Discuss any questions, concerns, or side effects you may be experiencing, and work together to address them.

10. **Patient Education:**

- Stay informed about your specific cancer type, potential late effects of treatment, and recommended follow-up care. Knowledge empowers you to actively participate in your ongoing health management.

11. **Genetic Counseling:**

- For individuals with a hereditary cancer predisposition, genetic counseling may be beneficial. Understanding your genetic risk can guide ongoing surveillance and risk management.

12. **Rehabilitation Services:**

- If you experienced physical challenges during treatment, consider rehabilitation services such as physical therapy or occupational therapy to support your recovery.

13. **Dental Health:**

- Pay attention to dental health, as certain cancer treatments may have long-term effects on oral health. Schedule regular dental check-ups and inform your dentist about your cancer history.

14. **Financial Considerations:**

- Address any financial considerations related to follow-up care, including insurance coverage, co-pays, and potential out-of-pocket expenses. Consult financial assistance resources if needed.

15. **Quality of Life Assessments:**

- Periodic assessments of your quality of life, including factors like pain, fatigue, and overall well-being, can help tailor ongoing support and interventions to enhance your daily life.

Celebrating Milestones and Achievements: Acknowledging Triumphs in the Cancer Journey

Celebrating milestones and achievements is an essential aspect of the cancer journey, offering moments of reflection, resilience, and triumph. Recognizing and commemorating these milestones not only honors the individual's strength but also provides a source of motivation and inspiration for the future. Here are strategies for celebrating milestones and achievements throughout the cancer journey:

Acknowledging Personal Milestones

Strategies:

- Reflection Rituals: Create personal rituals for reflection, such as journaling, to acknowledge and celebrate milestones, both big and small.
- Gratitude Practice: Cultivate a gratitude practice, expressing thanks for the progress made, supportive relationships, and personal growth experienced during the journey.

Commemorating Treatment Milestones

Strategies:

- Treatment Completion Ceremonies: Organize a treatment completion ceremony or symbolic event to mark the end of a particular phase of treatment, emphasizing resilience and moving forward.
- Artistic Expression: Use artistic expression, such as creating art or writing, to commemorate treatment milestones, capturing emotions and experiences visually or through words.

Sharing Achievements with Loved Ones

Strategies:

- Celebratory Gatherings: Arrange celebratory gatherings with friends and family to share achievements, fostering a sense of community and support.
- Personalized Celebrations: Tailor celebrations to personal preferences, whether it's a small intimate gathering or a larger event with loved ones.

Creating a Milestone Journal

Strategies:

- Milestone Journaling: Maintain a milestone journal to document accomplishments, challenges overcome, and personal growth throughout the cancer journey.
- Visual Representations: Incorporate visual representations, such as drawings or collages, to accompany written reflections in the milestone journal.

Setting and Recognizing Personal Goals

Strategies:

- Goal Setting: Set achievable personal goals and milestones, celebrating each accomplishment along the way.
- Self-Affirmations: Incorporate positive self-affirmations to recognize personal strengths and capabilities, reinforcing a sense of empowerment.

Creating Symbolic Tokens

Strategies:

- Symbolic Tokens: Create or acquire symbolic tokens, such as jewelry or artwork, representing milestones and achievements to serve as tangible reminders of strength and resilience.
- Customized Memorabilia: Design customized memorabilia, like a scrapbook or shadow box, containing items that symbolize milestones and triumphs in the cancer journey.

Organizing Surprise Celebrations

Strategies:

- Surprise Celebrations: Organize surprise celebrations planned by friends or family, bringing an element of joy and spontaneity to milestone acknowledgment.
- Theme-Based Events: Consider theme-based surprise events, aligning with personal interests or hobbies, to make the celebration extra special.

Connecting with Support Groups

Strategies:

- Support Group Celebrations: Celebrate milestones within support groups, where individuals share similar experiences, fostering a sense of camaraderie and encouragement.
- Virtual Celebrations: Utilize virtual platforms to connect with support groups and celebrate achievements together, overcoming geographical barriers.

Incorporating Humor and Lightness

Strategies:

- Humorous Celebrations: Infuse humor into milestone celebrations, finding lightness in moments and using laughter as a means of resilience.
- Comedic Events: Consider organizing comedic events or activities that bring joy and laughter, creating a positive and uplifting atmosphere.

Involving Healthcare Team in Celebrations

Strategies:

- Expressing Gratitude: Express gratitude to the healthcare team by involving them in milestone celebrations, acknowledging their role in the journey.
- Healthcare Team Recognition: Create certificates or small tokens of appreciation for healthcare professionals who have played a significant role in achieving milestones.

Planning Future Aspirations

Strategies:

- Future Aspiration Discussions: Engage in discussions about future aspirations and goals, using milestones as stepping stones toward new endeavors.
- Vision Board Creation: Develop a vision board that visually represents future aspirations and serves as a source of motivation and inspiration.

Commemorative Art and Creativity

Strategies:

- Artistic Commemoration: Collaborate with artists or engage in creative projects to create commemorative art pieces that represent the cancer journey and celebrate triumphs.
- Art Exhibitions or Showcases: Organize art exhibitions or showcases to share the creations with a wider audience, fostering a sense of community.

Community Acknowledgment and Recognition

Strategies:

- Community Acknowledgment: Engage with local communities or organizations to receive acknowledgment and recognition for milestones achieved, promoting awareness and understanding.
- Public Celebrations: Consider participating in public celebrations or events that highlight achievements, providing inspiration to others facing similar challenges.

Gratitude and Giving Back

Strategies:

- Giving Back: Give back to the community or support causes related to cancer awareness, transforming personal achievements into opportunities for positive impact.
- Gratitude Initiatives: Initiate gratitude initiatives, expressing thanks to those who have contributed to the journey, including healthcare professionals, caregivers, and support networks.

Annual Reflection and Celebration Day

Strategies:

- Annual Reflection Day: Designate an annual day for reflection and celebration, taking time to review accomplishments, express gratitude, and set intentions for the future.
- Personalized Rituals: Establish personalized rituals or traditions for the annual reflection day, making it a meaningful and cherished occasion.

Chapter 9: Resources and Further Reading: Navigating the Cancer Journey for Moms

General Cancer Resources

Websites:

- American Cancer Society
- National Cancer Institute
- Cancer.Net

Books:

- "The Emperor of All Maladies: A Biography of Cancer" by Siddhartha Mukherjee
- "When Breath Becomes Air" by Paul Kalanithi
- "Being Mortal: Medicine and What Matters in the End" by Atul Gawande

Support for Moms with Cancer

Websites:

- CancerCare - Helping You and Your Loved Ones
- Living Beyond Breast Cancer
- National Coalition for Cancer Survivorship

Books:

- "Crazy Sexy Cancer Tips" by Kris Carr
- "Dear Friend, Letters of Encouragement, Humor, and Love for Women with Breast Cancer" by Gina L. Mulligan

Emotional Support and Mental Health Resources

Websites:

- Cancer Support Community
- National Alliance on Mental Illness (NAMI)

Books:

- "Radical Remission: Surviving Cancer Against All Odds" by Kelly A. Turner
- "The Mindful Path to Self-Compassion: Freeing Yourself from Destructive Thoughts and Emotions" by Christopher K. Germer

Parenting and Cancer Resources

Websites:

- Cancer and Careers - Balancing Work and Cancer
- American Cancer Society - Children Diagnosed with Cancer

Books:

- "Cancer Mom: Hearing God in an Unknown Journey" by Kristi P. Hugstad
- "The Two-Step: The Dance Towards Intimacy After Divorce or Death" by Eileen R. Borris

Practical and Financial Resources

Websites:

- Patient Advocate Foundation
- Cancer Financial Assistance Coalition

Books:

- "Navigating Your Federal Retirement: Your Successful Passage into Financial Freedom" by Tammy Flanagan
- "The Total Money Makeover: A Proven Plan for Financial Fitness" by Dave Ramsey

Wellness and Self-Care Resources

Websites:

- LIVESTRONG Foundation - Cancer Support for the Whole Family
- Integrative Oncology Essentials

Books:

- "Anti-Cancer: A New Way of Life" by David Servan-Schreiber
- "The Cancer-Fighting Kitchen: Nourishing, Big-Flavor Recipes for Cancer Treatment and Recovery" by Rebecca Katz

Survivorship and Life After Cancer Resources

Websites:

- Cancer Survivorship: Next Steps for Patients and Their Families
- National Cancer Survivorship Resource Center

Books:

- "A Cancer Survivor's Almanac: Charting Your Journey" by Barbara Hoffman
- "After Cancer Care: The Definitive Self-Care Guide to Getting and Staying Well for Patients After Cancer" by Gerald M. Lemole, Pallav K. Mehta, and Dwight L. McKee

Caregiver Support Resources

Websites:

- Family Caregiver Alliance
- CancerCare - For Caregivers

Books:

- "The Caregiving Wife's Handbook: Caring for Your Seriously Ill Husband, Caring for Yourself" by Diana B. Denholm
- "The 36-Hour Day: A Family Guide to Caring for People Who Have Alzheimer's Disease, Other Dementias, and Memory Loss" by Nancy L. Mace and Peter V. Rabins

Community and Peer Support Resources

Websites:

- Smart Patients - Cancer Forums
- Cancer Support Community - Online Support Groups

Books:

- "Living with Cancer: A Step-by-Step Guide for Coping Medically and Emotionally with a Serious Diagnosis" by Vicki A. Jackson, David P. Ryan, and Michelle D. Seaton
- "Supportive Cancer Care: The Complete Guide for Patients and Their Families" by Ernest H. Rosenbaum and Isadora R. Rosenbaum

Advocacy and Education Resources

Websites:

- National Patient Advocate Foundation
- American Cancer Society - Cancer Action Network

Books:

- "Advocacy Heals U: 15 Keys to Fast Track Results and Emotional Fulfillment" by Joni Aldrich
- "The Cancer Revolution: A Groundbreaking Program to Reverse and Prevent Cancer" by Leigh Erin Connealy

Nutrition and Wellness Resources

Websites:

- American Institute for Cancer Research - Nutrition and Cancer
- NutritionFacts.org

Books:

- "Eat to Beat Disease: The New Science of How Your Body Can Heal Itself" by William W. Li
- "The Plant-Based Solution: America's Healthy Heart Doc's Plan to Power Your Health" by Joel K. Kahn

Conclusion: Embracing Resilience and Hope on the Cancer Journey for Moms

The cancer journey for moms is a profound and challenging path, marked by a complex interplay of emotions, decisions, and adaptations. As we conclude this comprehensive guide, it's essential to reflect on the resilience, strength, and hope that characterize the experiences of mothers facing cancer.

The journey encompasses a range of topics, from the initial shock of diagnosis to the complexities of treatment decisions, emotional well-being, and life after cancer. Throughout each stage, the importance of a robust support system, including healthcare professionals, family, and friends, emerges as a consistent theme.

Key Takeaways:

Empowerment through Knowledge: Understanding the nuances of cancer, its types, causes, and treatment options empowers moms to actively engage in decision-making and advocate for their well-being.

Holistic Support: Beyond medical interventions, emotional, practical, and financial support is crucial. Recognizing and addressing the emotional impact, managing practical matters, and navigating healthcare systems collectively contribute to holistic well-being.

Treatment Decision-Making: The diagnostic and treatment phases involve complex decision-making. From surgery and chemotherapy to radiation, moms navigate a range of treatments with the guidance of healthcare professionals.

Emotional Resilience: Coping with the emotional impact of cancer is a central aspect of the journey. Moms must explore strategies to cope with the initial diagnosis, communicate with family, and manage their emotional well-being throughout treatment.

Practical Considerations: Navigating practical matters, including financial considerations, balancing work, and building a support network, ensures that moms can focus on their health and well-being.

Life After Cancer: The transition to life after treatment marks a new beginning. Celebrating milestones, managing survivorship, and addressing physical and emotional well-being contribute to a fulfilling post-cancer life.

Resources and Support: A wealth of resources, from general cancer organizations to specialized support for moms, provides information, assistance, and a sense of community. Utilizing these resources ensures a well-rounded approach to navigating the cancer journey.

In the face of challenges, the strength of moms shines through. The love, resilience, and hope that define motherhood become powerful forces in overcoming the obstacles presented by cancer. As we conclude, it's essential to recognize that the journey doesn't end with cancer; rather, it transforms into a story of survival, strength, and the pursuit of a fulfilling life beyond the diagnosis.

Reflecting on the Cancer Journey: A Personal and Collective Journey of Resilience

As we pause to reflect on the profound and transformative experience of the cancer journey, it is a moment to honor the resilience, courage, and strength that characterize this formidable odyssey. Each step, from the initial shock of diagnosis to the challenges of treatment and the emergence into life after cancer, is marked by a tapestry of emotions, decisions, and unwavering hope.

1. The Power of Knowledge:

- *Empowerment through Understanding:* Knowledge is a formidable ally in the face of uncertainty. Understanding the intricacies of cancer, its varied forms, and the available treatment options empowers individuals to make informed decisions and actively participate in their healthcare journey.

2. Emotional Landscape:

- *Navigating the Depths of Emotion:* The emotional impact of a cancer diagnosis is profound. From the initial shock to the ongoing challenges of treatment, individuals embark on a journey that requires resilience and a supportive network. Recognizing and addressing the emotional landscape is a vital aspect of healing.

3. Treatment Decisions and Resilience:

- *Complex Decision-Making:* The journey through diagnosis, treatment options, and decisions regarding surgery, chemotherapy, or radiation is a complex tapestry. In the midst of medical choices, resilience becomes a guiding force, navigating individuals through the challenges with strength and determination.

4. Holistic Well-Being:

- *Beyond Medical Interventions:* The cancer journey extends beyond medical interventions, encompassing the holistic well-being of individuals. Managing practical matters, navigating healthcare systems, and building a robust support system contribute to a comprehensive approach to health and recovery.

5. Celebration of Milestones:

- *Triumphs Along the Way:* Celebrating milestones, both big and small, becomes a poignant aspect of the journey. Whether completing a phase of treatment or embracing life after cancer, acknowledging triumphs fosters a sense of accomplishment and resilience.

6. Community and Support:

- *Strength in Unity:* The support of a community, including healthcare professionals, family, friends, and fellow survivors, becomes a lifeline. Building a network that understands the challenges and celebrates the victories creates an environment of shared strength and solidarity.

7. Life After Cancer:

- *A New Beginning:* Life after cancer marks a profound transition, requiring adjustment and a focus on well-being. Survivorship is not just about physical recovery but also about embracing the opportunities for a renewed and fulfilling life.

8. Reflection and Gratitude:

- *Acknowledging the Journey:* Taking moments for reflection allows individuals to acknowledge the journey they have traversed. Expressing gratitude for the support received, the lessons learned, and the strength discovered along the way becomes a cathartic process.

9. Shared Narratives:

- *Collective Wisdom:* The cancer journey is a collective narrative of strength, hope, and shared experiences. Each individual's story contributes to a broader tapestry of resilience, offering insights and inspiration to others navigating similar paths.

10. The Unseen Heroes:

- *Caregivers and Healthcare Professionals:* Behind every individual on the cancer journey stand unseen heroes—dedicated caregivers and healthcare professionals. Their compassion, expertise, and unwavering support play a pivotal role in the healing process.

In reflecting on the cancer journey, it is crucial to recognize that the path is not linear. It is marked by peaks of triumph and valleys of challenge. Yet, within each ebb and flow, there exists a reservoir of strength that transcends the physical realm. It is a testament to the human spirit—a spirit that can endure, learn, and emerge stronger.

Moving Forward with Hope: Navigating the Post-Cancer Horizon

As we stand at the threshold of the post-cancer horizon, the journey forward is imbued with a sense of hope, renewal, and the promise of new beginnings. Moving beyond the shadows of diagnosis and treatment, individuals emerge as survivors, resilient and equipped with the wisdom gained from the challenges faced. Here are key considerations for moving forward with hope:

1. Cultivating a Renewed Perspective:

- Embrace a mindset of renewal and transformation. Recognize the strength that has been unearthed during the journey and view life through a lens of gratitude and resilience.

2. Prioritizing Self-Care:

- Self-care remains paramount in the post-cancer phase. Prioritize physical, emotional, and mental well-being, incorporating practices that nourish and rejuvenate the body and spirit.

3. Setting Realistic Goals:

- Establish realistic and achievable goals for the future. Whether they pertain to personal growth, relationships, or professional aspirations, setting milestones provides a roadmap for the journey ahead.

4. Rebuilding Relationships:

- Strengthen connections with loved ones and rebuild relationships that may have been affected during the cancer journey. Open communication fosters understanding and a renewed sense of closeness.

5. Exploring New Possibilities:

- The post-cancer horizon is a canvas for exploration. Consider pursuing new interests, hobbies, or activities that align with personal passions and aspirations.

6. Continuing Follow-Up Care:

- Regular follow-up care and health surveillance are essential components of post-cancer life. Work closely with healthcare professionals to monitor health and address any concerns promptly.

7. Celebrating Milestones:

- Continue to celebrate milestones, both large and small. Acknowledge achievements and use them as a source of motivation for the ongoing journey.

8. Engaging in Advocacy:

- Channel the experiences gained during the cancer journey into advocacy efforts. Raise awareness, share insights, and contribute to the broader conversation surrounding cancer awareness and survivorship.

9. Supporting Others:

- Extend support to those currently navigating the challenges of a cancer diagnosis. Share experiences, provide encouragement, and offer insights that may serve as beacons of hope for others.

10. Nurturing Emotional Resilience:

- Emotional well-being remains a focal point. Nurture emotional resilience by engaging in practices such as mindfulness, counseling, or support groups that foster a sense of balance and self-awareness.

11. Exploring New Beginnings:

- Embrace the concept of new beginnings. Whether it involves a career change, relocation, or a fresh approach to life, view the post-cancer horizon as an opportunity for growth and exploration.

12. Integrating Lessons Learned:

- Reflect on the lessons learned during the cancer journey and integrate them into daily life. These lessons become the foundation for a mindful and purposeful approach to living.

13. Fostering a Sense of Community:

- Engage with survivorship communities and support networks. Sharing experiences and insights creates a sense of belonging and reinforces the collective strength of survivors.

14. Gratitude and Reflection:

- Practice gratitude for the journey, acknowledging the strength and support that accompanied each step. Reflect on the transformative nature of the experience and the growth that has unfolded.

15. Embracing the Gift of Today:

- Live in the present moment, savoring the gift of today. Approach each day with a sense of gratitude, hope, and an appreciation for the beauty inherent in life.

Glossary: Understanding Key Terms in the Cancer Journey for Moms

As individuals navigate the complex landscape of the cancer journey, it is helpful to have a grasp of key terms and terminology. This glossary provides definitions to aid in understanding various aspects of the cancer experience:

Biopsy:
- The removal and examination of a small tissue sample to diagnose or rule out the presence of cancer.

Chemotherapy:
- A treatment method that uses drugs to kill or slow the growth of cancer cells.

Diagnosis:
- The identification and determination of the nature of a disease or condition, such as cancer.

Early Detection:
- The identification of cancer at an early, more treatable stage through screening or other diagnostic methods.

Holistic Care:
- Comprehensive care that addresses not only the physical aspects of cancer but also emotional, social, and spiritual well-being.

Mammogram:
- An X-ray of the breast used for screening and diagnosing breast cancer.

Oncologist:
- A medical doctor who specializes in the diagnosis and treatment of cancer.

Radiation Therapy:
- The use of high doses of radiation to kill or damage cancer cells.

Support Groups:
- Gatherings of individuals facing similar challenges, providing emotional support, shared experiences, and information.

Survivorship:
- The period after cancer treatment when individuals focus on recovery, well-being, and maintaining a healthy lifestyle.

Tumor:
- An abnormal mass of tissue that may be benign (non-cancerous) or malignant (cancerous).

Wellness:
- An overall state of well-being that involves a balance of physical, mental, and social health.

Clinical Trial:
- Research studies that involve human participants, designed to test new treatments or interventions.

Caregiver:
- An individual, often a family member or friend, who provides support and assistance to someone facing a health challenge, such as cancer.

Metastasis:
- The spread of cancer cells from the original site to other parts of the body.

Pathology:
- The branch of medicine that studies the nature and causes of diseases, including examining tissues and cells for diagnosis.

Screening:
- Testing or examination to identify a disease, such as cancer, in its early stages before symptoms appear.

Remission:
- The partial or complete disappearance of signs and symptoms of cancer, indicating a response to treatment.

Cancer Support Community:
- An organization providing support, education, and resources for individuals and families affected by cancer.

Integrative Therapies:

- Complementary approaches, such as acupuncture, massage, or mindfulness, used alongside conventional cancer treatments to enhance well-being.

Disclaimer: This Guide is Not Medical Advice

The information provided in this guide on the cancer journey for moms is intended for general informational purposes only. It is not a substitute for professional medical advice, diagnosis, or treatment. Always seek the advice of your physician or other qualified healthcare providers with any questions you may have regarding a medical condition.

The content within this guide is based on general knowledge and does not account for individual health circumstances. Each person's cancer journey is unique, and medical decisions should be tailored to specific needs and guided by healthcare professionals.

While efforts have been made to ensure the accuracy and completeness of the information presented, it is subject to change as new medical advancements and research emerge. The author and publisher are not responsible for any errors or omissions or for any consequences arising from the use of the information provided in this guide.

Readers are encouraged to consult with their healthcare providers for personalized advice, diagnosis, or treatment plans. The goal of this guide is to offer support, information, and insights into various aspects of the cancer journey, but it should not be considered a substitute for professional medical guidance.